THE HUMAN FACE OF PANDEMICS

THE HUMAN FACE OF PANDEMICS

EMOTION, MEANING, AND MISSED PREVENTION IN PANDEMIC LIFE

Carlo Lazzari • Jon Rees •
Yitka Graham • Rebecca Owens

First published in 2026 by Libri Publishing

ISBN 978-1-911451-49-5 paperback
ISBN 978-1-911451-60-0 hardback

A CIP catalogue record for this book is available from
The British Library

Cover and design by Carnegie Book Production

Libri Publishing
Brunel House
Volunteer Way
Faringdon
Oxfordshire
SN7 7YR

Tel: +44 (0)845 873 3837

www.libripublishing.co.uk

Contents

Definition of terms

Covid19 (COVID-19): An infectious disease caused by the coronavirus SARSCoV2. It primarily affects the respiratory system but can involve multiple organs. Clinical presentations range from asymptomatic to severe, and the disease triggered the global pandemic beginning in 2020.

HIV (Human Immunodeficiency Virus): A virus that targets and progressively damages the immune system, especially CD4 (Thelper) cells. It is transmitted through specific bodily fluids such as blood, semen, vaginal secretions, and breast milk.

AIDS (Acquired Immunodeficiency Syndrome): The advanced stage of untreated HIV infection, defined by severe immune suppression and the presence of opportunistic infections or certain cancers.

Virus: A microscopic infectious agent that requires a living host cell to replicate. Viruses infect organisms across all domains of life, including humans, animals, plants, and bacteria.

Pandemic: A large-scale outbreak of a disease that spreads across multiple countries or continents, affecting a substantial proportion of the population. Defined by geographic spread rather than severity.

Epidemic: A sudden increase in the number of cases of a disease above what is usually expected in a specific region or population.

Phenomenology: A philosophical approach that examines lived experience as it is consciously perceived, aiming to reveal the essential structures of consciousness without imposing external theories.

Ontology: The branch of philosophy concerned with the nature of being and existence. It explores the entities that exist, how they can be categorised, and the relationships between them.

Epistemology: The study of knowledge—its nature, sources, justification, and limits. It investigates how beliefs become knowledge and how humans acquire, validate, and interpret information.

Axiology: The philosophical study of value, encompassing ethics (moral value) and aesthetics (value of beauty). It examines what is considered good, meaningful, or worthwhile.

Syndrome of Samos: A concept introduced by Carlo Lazzari describing a form of *pathophilia* in which individuals consciously or unconsciously reject protective health behaviours during pandemics. It reflects a psychological and existential stance where transmissible diseases do not prompt the expected health behaviours, undermining personal and public health efforts.

CHAPTER 1

Introduction

Introduction

The World Health Organization (2021) defines a pandemic as "an epidemic occurring worldwide, or over a vast area, crossing international boundaries and usually affecting a large number of people," without reference to immunity, virology, or disease severity. Similarly, the Merriam-Webster Dictionary Online (2025) defines a pandemic as an event "occurring over a wide geographic area (such as multiple countries or continents) and typically affecting a significant proportion of the population," without specifying bacterial or viral causes. The Cambridge Dictionary Online (2025a) broadens the scope to include diseases affecting nearly all members of a group—humans, animals, or plants—across a large area.

These definitions emphasise scale and reach rather than biological specifics. According to the United States Centers for Disease Control and Prevention (CDC), an outbreak is "when an illness happens in unexpectedly high numbers. It may stay in one area or extend more widely. An outbreak can last days or years" (CDC, 2024). In the context of a pandemic, such outbreaks—occurring as acute, localised surges within the broader global spread—are often described as pandemic outbursts. These outbreaks usually reflect sudden increases in transmission driven by behavioural, environmental, or policy-related factors and may require targeted public health interventions to prevent wider escalation.

In social science, the theoretical framing of pandemics is shaped by ontology, epistemology, and axiology. Ontology examines the nature of reality, questioning what exists and how constructs such as identity, power, and institutions are formed. Positivist perspectives hold that truth is objective, whereas constructivist perspectives emphasise socially constructed meaning (Crotty, 1998; Guba and Lincoln, 1994). Epistemology concerns how knowledge is acquired and validated, guiding methodological choices between positivist approaches that prioritise measurable data and interpretivist approaches that highlight subjective understanding and co-constructed meaning (Creswell and Poth, 2018; Cohen, Manion, and Morrison, 2018). Axiology addresses the ethical and value-based aspects of research, recognising that inquiry is never neutral. It must consider what is worth studying and how ethical principles influence the process—especially in contexts involving human participants and social justice (Guba and Lincoln, 1994; Scotland, 2012). During pandemics, these conceptual domains shape how individuals perceive threats, engage with information, and make ethical choices. They offer a comprehensive view of diverse public responses to crises, uncertainty, and health interventions.

Pandemics produce complex and lasting impacts across populations, including psychological distress, legal disruptions, behavioural changes, and existential confusion. When our research into Covid-19 began on 12 April 2020, the United Kingdom had reported approximately 133,495 confirmed cases and 18,100 deaths, while global figures stood at 2,628,527 cases and over 183,424 deaths (Public Health England, 2020). As of mid-October 2025, Covid-19 activity in the UK remains moderate, with 2,618 confirmed cases reported in the most recent week—a 20.2% decrease from the previous period—while deaths increased by 41% to 141 and hospital admissions rose by 9.7% to 2,077. The test positivity rate is currently 11.8%, indicating ongoing community transmission. Although case numbers are decreasing, the simultaneous rise in deaths and hospital admissions highlights the need for continued public health vigilance, especially as influenza activity rises among children and respiratory syncytial virus circulates at typical levels (UK Health Security Agency, 2025).

Although these figures are concerning, they only partially capture the extent of societal upheaval. As Watts (1999) observed, public anxiety during epidemics stems not only from suffering and death but also from the broader collapse of civilisational norms. The rapid spread of Covid-19 prompted urgent reflection within the public and mental health sectors on its direct and indirect physical, social, and emotional effects on individuals and communities. Those who are frail, chronically ill, socially isolated, or otherwise vulnerable face increased risks—not only from the virus itself but also from the psychological and systemic impacts of prolonged and recurring existential crises during pandemics. In some cases, underlying health behaviours may weaken individuals' mental or physical resilience, undermine well-being, and necessitate health actions during pandemics, such as prioritising others' safety or adopting protective measures (Lazzari and Masino, 2015). This poses significant challenges for implementing strategies to prevent social contagion. Individuals with limited emotional or cognitive resilience may be more severely affected by viral outbreaks, and emotional vulnerability and difficulty in endorsing primary prevention further hamper public health efforts.

Individuals with heightened psychological sensitivity may struggle to grasp abstract concepts such as contagion, self-preservation, and communal responsibility. Deep-seated beliefs, cultural biases, and habitual behaviours can impede understanding of how transmissible diseases affect personal and collective well-being. Our research also highlights widespread disruptions in education and workplaces, including the suspension and reorganisation of university programmes, the cancellation of face-to-face lectures and examinations, and the redefinition of interprofessional collaboration under emergency protocols. These changes highlight the pandemic's impact on institutional, epistemic, and operational frameworks and emphasise the need for not only biomedical solutions but also phenomenological insights into how populations experience, interpret, and emotionally manage pandemics. In this book, we aim to distil, from our existing work, a clear set of theoretical frameworks—ranging from middle-range to grand theories—that examine the psychological, sociological, and biological dimensions of pandemics, with particular emphasis on the lived experiences and systemic responses observed during the AIDS and

Covid-19 crises. Through empirical research and workplace learning, we seek to synthesise policy recommendations and preventative strategies to strengthen primary prevention for future pandemics. Our perspective is further informed by our roles as senior healthcare practitioners within the United Kingdom's National Health Service (NHS) and in academia, supported by postgraduate training and clinical expertise in infectious diseases, psychology, and public health.

Our engagement studies on the spread of pandemics began during specialised training in HIV/AIDS psychiatry and later expanded to include Covid-19. In both contexts, we identified distinct cognitive and emotional patterns in how populations respond to the threat of transmissible diseases. These insights, drawn from longitudinal research and clinical practice, inform our theoretical and practical advice on the impact of pandemics and on how to prevent them. Through ongoing publications, we have contributed to the literature on the psychosocial aspects of infectious diseases and health-related behaviours, tracking their development over time. Although this project partly reflects recent findings on Covid-19, its conceptual framework is grounded in a broader trajectory of inquiry that began with the AIDS pandemic and includes other transmissible conditions referred to here as 'pandemics'.

Pandemics are not merely biological disruptions but complex crises that raise questions about shared meanings, ethics, and knowledge. The Covid-19 pandemic exposed tensions between scientific authority, moral judgement, and behavioural compliance, rooted in contested ideas of expertise, agency, and civic duty. Douglas (2009) argues that scientific reasoning is linked to moral values, particularly when public health policies affect daily life, whereas Broadbent (2013; 2020; 2022) criticises strict evidence hierarchies and advocates a pluralistic, context-sensitive epistemology. Phenomenological perspectives—such as Carel's (2018; 2020) concept of embodied disruption and Svenaeus's (2001) view of illness as unhomelike being-in-the-world—demonstrate how pandemics fracture identity and evoke existential uncertainty. Lazzari, Gandolfi Colleoni, and Trallo (1996) propose a framework that integrates ontology, epistemology, and axiology to show how pandemics distort reasoning and moral coherence. Responses to pandemics at the individual, organisational, and policy levels are often shaped by emotional resilience, institutional trust, and cultural norms, with misinformation and symbolic acts influencing risk perception and ethical choices (Guzman et al., 2023; Caperon, Saville, and Ahern, 2022).

Public health ethics, supported by relational and conceptual bioethics, advocate emotionally intelligent, solidarity-driven responses grounded in normative analysis. Dewey's pragmatism (1925; 1927; 1939) and Thompson and Upshur's (2017) work frame pandemics as moral and epistemic events rather than merely scientific challenges. We adopt a conceptual-analytical approach to examine how pandemics transform societal notions of truth, trust, and responsibility, combining conceptual investigation with phenomenological analysis to explore the interdependence of cognition, culture, and health governance. Phenomenology, both as a conceptual tradition and as a research method, investigates the structure of lived experience from a first-person perspective (Churchill, 2014), examining how perception, emotion, embodiment, and intentionality shape experience. Husserl (1931) promoted a "return to the things themselves," introducing concepts such as epoché and phenomenological reduction to reveal the essential structures of consciousness. Merleau-Ponty (1962) expanded on this by emphasising the embodied nature of perception, arguing that the body is an active medium through which the world is disclosed, thereby challenging Cartesian dualism and recasting subjectivity as inherently corporeal and relational (Stewart and Mikunas, 1974). This embodied focus has shaped contemporary uses of phenomenology across psychology, cognitive science, health ethics, and organisational studies, offering a nuanced lens for understanding lived reality.

Hence, we adopt a phenomenological approach to understanding pandemic-related health behaviours, focusing on how individuals experience and interpret public health crises within their lived realities. Rather than relying on empirical metrics or clinical outcomes, we examine how people respond emotionally and cognitively to preventive measures such as mask-wearing, social distancing, and isolation. As Erciyes (2019) explains, phenomenology—rooted in the works of Husserl, Heidegger, and Merleau-Ponty—prioritises the first-person perspective, making it particularly suited to examining how individuals create meaning in conditions of uncertainty. Health behaviours during pandemics are not merely acts of compliance or resistance; they are embodied expressions shaped by anxiety, ethical reasoning, and evolving perceptions of self and community. For example, Zahavi and Szanto (2023) show that mask-wearing can evoke a range of emotional responses—from protection and solidarity to alienation and discomfort—depending on one's cultural and interpersonal context.

Similarly, Liu and Liu (2021), in their phenomenological account of hospitalised Covid-19 patients, show that isolation can lead to deep emotional distress, temporal disorientation, and existential unease. These experiences illustrate how individuals integrate health behaviours into personal narratives, sense-making, and moral frameworks. For example, during pandemic lockdowns, time may feel suspended, and public spaces can take on symbolic meanings, either as dangerous sites or places of longing. Butler (2022) describes this shift as a reorientation of everyday meaning, in which disruption prompts reflection on vulnerability, interdependence, and the fragility of social bonds. From this perspective, health behaviour is not simply a biological necessity or a sociological trend; it is a profoundly human process of creating meaning. A phenomenological approach, therefore, provides a strong tool for understanding how individuals manage the moral tensions between collective responsibility and personal autonomy, especially in the context of prevention during public health crises.

Phenomenology, ontology, epistemology, and axiology of pandemics

Phenomenological analysis offers a crucial perspective on pandemic-related phenomena by emphasising the lived experiences of individuals and communities in the contexts of prevention, control, and viral dissemination. Rather than viewing health behaviours solely as rational responses to biomedical information, phenomenology examines how illness, risk, and preventive measures are interpreted through embodied, emotional, and symbolic dimensions within individuals (Svenaeus, 2001). Public health interventions are thus not merely objective facts but are filtered through personal histories, cultural narratives, and existential perspectives. Emotional states such as vulnerability, shame, and alienation can significantly shape health responses to actions such as vaccination or quarantine, often resulting in behaviours that diverge from those anticipated by epidemiologists and policymakers (Lazzari, Gandolfi Colleoni, and Trallo, 1996). Phenomenology challenges the assumption that increased knowledge automatically leads to behavioural change; instead, it highlights the gap between awareness and action, where denial, fatalism, and relational dynamics may supersede self-protective instincts (Valli et al., 2002). The aestheticisation of risk—where danger is romanticised or symbolically accepted—further stresses the importance of culturally sensitive and psychologically informed public health strategies (Lazzari, Gandolfi Colleoni, and Trallo, 1996). Furthermore, by focusing on the subjective aspects of health behaviours, phenomenology explains why individuals might resist or reinterpret public health messages, even when risks are broadly recognised. Consequently, when integrated with epistemology, ontology, and axiology, phenomenology enhances our understanding of the human impact of pandemics. Epistemology critiques the dominance of statistical abstraction and advocates pluralistic knowledge systems that incorporate experiential and relational insights (Dupré and Leonelli, 2022). Ontology redefines pandemics as existential disruptions or states of estrangement rather than purely biological events (Svenaeus, 2001). Axiology stresses that health behaviours are influenced not only by risk assessments but also by values, desires, and moral negotiations (Thompson and Upshur, 2017). Collectively, these conceptual frameworks affirm that an effective response to pandemics must be ethically reflective, emotionally resonant, and grounded in the complexity of human experience.

Major stakeholders and beneficiaries of our research include the general population, who gain a deeper understanding of how pandemics influence individual health behaviours and how these behaviours can be modified to reduce risk; mental health services, which gain insights to better prepare for and respond to the psychological and systemic consequences of current and future pandemics; and public health organisations—both government and non-government—that can refine prevention strategies and more effectively target vulnerable groups by incorporating biopsychosocial insights into their campaigns and by strengthening primary prevention frameworks. The selected public works supporting this book, together with reflective analyses from our broader research portfolio, address several critical challenges that emerge during pandemics: first, ontological disruption and cognitive decline, in which we examine how social isolation reshapes the experience of self and relational identity, and how disrupted social networks affect cognitive coherence, identity continuity, and neuropsychological resilience; second, the epistemic traits of high diffusers, identifying the psychological and epistemological characteristics of individuals who widely disseminate information or contagion, including their belief systems, risk perception, and moral reasoning under uncertainty; third, axiological shifts in health behaviours across historical pandemics, interpreting emergent behaviours as reflections of changing societal values, ethical norms, and survival strategies, with parallels to contemporary responses to Covid-19 and other outbreaks; fourth, transformations in learning and knowledge systems post-Covid-19, analysing how pandemics reconfigure educational epistemologies, including digital pedagogy, learner autonomy, and the integration of uncertainty into curriculum design and knowledge validation; fifth, alleviating mental health burdens in non-clinical populations by developing ethically grounded, value-sensitive interventions to foster resilience, meaning-making, and community-based psychological support; sixth, understanding and managing extremes of behaviour under pandemic threats, investigating ontological destabilisation and axiological polarisation that fuel denialism, hoarding, and aggression, and proposing integrative models for psychosocial containment and ethical governance; and seventh, reimagining primary prevention through a phenomenological lens, enhancing public health strategies by embedding epistemic humility, ethical pluralism, and ontological sensitivity into messaging, stakeholder engagement, and anticipatory care models.

Methodologies and methods in pandemic research

Most of our scholarly contributions to pandemic studies employed a naturalistic, qualitative, and inductive methodology to explore key themes across the psychological, sociological, and biological dimensions of pandemics, with particular focus on Covid-19 and AIDS. Among these, one systematic review examined the cognitive consequences of social isolation in adult populations, while a separate quantitative study assessed the structural impact of Covid-19 on higher education systems. Our methodological approach to uncovering new facts about pandemics is interpretive, adopting an inductive-qualitative framework to synthesise middle-range and grand theories derived from our research, consistent with a Grounded Theory approach.

As a desk-based synthesis, we do not introduce new empirical data but draw on our existing research to craft a reflective narrative rooted in our settings, practice, and daily experiences during pandemic scenarios. Furthermore, from a researcher-practitioner perspective, we aimed to identify actionable insights for policy development and to enhance pandemic prevention strategies. Through detailed descriptions of organisational experiences and tacit knowledge, we examined the theoretical development and practical significance of our findings. Ethical integrity remained central to this process, with careful attention to the responsible presentation of facts to avoid exposing vulnerable populations or institutions to unintended consequences that could undermine ongoing pandemic control efforts.

CHAPTER 2

Challenges and Impact of Pandemics

Ontology: What is real during a pandemic?

Ontology, the conceptual study of reality and the constitution of social phenomena (Lawson, 2012), plays a vital role in shaping how pandemics are understood and responded to. In the context of a pandemic, a positivist ontology holds that the virus, its transmission mechanisms, and its physiological effects are objectively tangible and measurable, existing independently of human perception. This ontological stance underpins biomedical models and epidemiological surveillance systems, which rely on empirical data to monitor infection rates, mortality, and intervention outcomes (Crotty, 1998; Guba and Lincoln, 1994). By contrast, a constructivist ontology regards reality as socially constructed, suggesting that individuals interpret the pandemic through cultural narratives, media representations, and personal experiences (Guba and Lincoln, 1994). For example, while some see Covid-19 as an urgent global health crisis requiring strict adherence to public health measures, others may regard it as exaggerated or politically manipulated, leading to different behavioural responses to prevention. This ontological divergence helps explain why public reactions to health mandates vary widely: each person responds to a different version of "reality" shaped by their own ontological assumptions.

Epistemology: How do we know what we know?

Epistemology, the study of how knowledge is acquired, interpreted, and validated (Crotty, 1998), plays a vital role in shaping public responses during pandemics. It shapes how individuals assess the credibility of information about the pandemic's nature, spread, and prevention, and decide whom or what to trust—be it scientific institutions, government bodies, or personal networks. A positivist epistemology prioritises objective, measurable data such as infection rates, vaccine efficacy, and transmission metrics, leading those who adopt this approach to rely heavily on official statistics and the consensus of scientific authorities (Creswell and Poth, 2018). Conversely, interpretivist epistemologies emphasise subjective understanding and the co-construction of meaning, prompting individuals to question dominant narratives and trust anecdotal accounts, community experiences, or alternative sources of information (Cohen, Manion, and Morrison, 2018). This epistemic divergence notably shapes public behaviour. For instance, decisions such as whether to accept vaccination, follow lockdown restrictions, or engage in preventive measures often depend on how individuals define "valid" knowledge and which scientific truths they endorse. Therefore, recognising these epistemological orientations is essential for designing inclusive and effective public health communication strategies that resonate across diverse belief systems and knowledge cultures.

Axiology: What do we value in a crisis?

Axiology, the study of values and ethics (Schwandt, 2007), plays a crucial role in shaping how individuals and societies respond to pandemics. It examines what people regard as essential, just, and morally acceptable, thereby influencing both personal behaviour and institutional decisions. During a health crisis, axiology guides moral reasoning, public debate, and policy development. For some, individual freedom (of thought and action) is vital, leading to adherence to or resistance against public health measures such as lockdowns, mask-wearing, or vaccination, which are perceived as infringements on personal autonomy. Others prioritise collective welfare, viewing compliance with health directives as a moral duty to protect vulnerable members of society.

These differing value systems often clash in public debates, revealing the ethical tensions underpinning pandemic governance. Researchers and policymakers also face complex moral dilemmas, such as balancing individual privacy with effective contact tracing or weighing economic stability against the need to protect public health (see Guba and Lincoln, 1994; Scotland, 2012). Axiology shows that pandemic-related behaviours are influenced not only by empirical data and fear but also by deeply held beliefs about justice, responsibility, and the common good.

When considered alongside ontology and epistemology, axiology completes a three-part framework for understanding pandemic behaviour. Ontology explains why people perceive different realities during pandemic events; epistemology clarifies how they determine what counts as credible knowledge to initiate or discontinue pandemic prevention measures; and axiology reveals the ethical principles that guide decisions to accept or reject recommendations for personal and social prevention. Recognising these conceptual foundations is crucial for developing public health strategies that are not only evidence-based but also ethically sound and culturally sensitive, thereby promoting greater empathy and cooperation during pandemic crises.

Phenomenology

In social science, phenomenology is a qualitative research method that explores and describes how individuals perceive and interpret everyday phenomena. Rooted in the ideas of Edmund Husserl and further developed by thinkers such as Martin Heidegger and Maurice Merleau-Ponty, phenomenology aims to uncover the essential nature of lived experience by deliberately bracketing preconceived theories and assumptions (Creswell and Poth, 2018).

This approach emphasises subjective perception, the construction of meaning, and the situational context of experiences, making it particularly effective for exploring complex human behaviours and emotional responses. In the context of pandemic-related health behaviours, phenomenology offers a vital perspective on how individuals interpret illness, risk, social isolation, and public health directives. Rather than relying solely on statistical data or predictive behavioural models, phenomenological inquiry engages with personal narratives, capturing how people respond emotionally to pandemic-related health behaviours, for example, by wearing masks, managing the psychological effects of lockdowns, and grappling with internal dilemmas about vaccination.

These insights illuminate the subtle, often unspoken factors that shape compliance, resistance, and adaptation during public health emergencies. By revealing these complexities, phenomenological research equips epidemiologists, policymakers, and health professionals with the tools to develop interventions that are not only evidence-based but also empathetic, culturally sensitive, and responsive to the lived experiences of diverse populations (Finlay, 2009; van Manen, 1990; Table 1).

Table 1: Summative table

Concept	Explanation	Application
Ontology:	Study of what is real; it explores the nature of reality during a pandemic. Positivist ontology regards the virus as objectively real, whereas constructivist ontology regards reality as socially constructed (e.g., conspiracy theories of viral dissemination).	Shapes pandemic responses: biomedical models rely on objective data, whereas public reactions vary according to individuals' perceptions of reality (e.g., compliance versus scepticism).
Epistemology:	Study of how we know what we know; examines how knowledge is acquired and validated—positivist epistemology values objective data, whereas interpretivist epistemology values subjective understanding.	Influences trust and behaviour: some rely on scientific data and authorities, while others rely on personal stories or alternative sources. Affects decisions such as vaccination uptake and adherence to health measures.
Axiology:	The study of values and ethics examines what individuals prioritise in a crisis. Some emphasise personal freedom, while others emphasise collective well-being.	Drives ethical decisions and public discourse: influences compliance with mandates, policymaking, and debates on privacy versus public health. Helps design morally resonant health strategies.

Concept	Explanation	Application
Phenomenology:	Study of lived experience; focuses on how individuals perceive and interpret everyday events. Emphasises subjective meaning and emotional responses.	Provides deep insight into personal experiences of pandemics. Helps to understand emotional responses to primary prevention measures, such as isolation, mask-wearing, and vaccination. Supports empathetic, culturally sensitive public health interventions. Provides deep insight into personal experiences of pandemics. Helps to understand emotional responses to primary prevention measures, such as isolation, mask-wearing, and vaccination. Supports empathetic, culturally sensitive public health interventions.

A Grounded Theory framework for understanding pandemic-health behaviours

Grounded Theory offers a robust and adaptable methodological framework for examining the psychological effects of pandemics, particularly in settings characterised by uncertainty, isolation, and systemic upheaval. Developed by Glaser and Strauss (1967), Grounded Theory is particularly effective at capturing emerging phenomena and facilitating the development of theory directly from individuals' lived experiences during public health crises. In our clinical research, this approach has been vital in identifying relational patterns between personal behavioural responses and broader sociopolitical factors.

Drawing on Strauss and Corbin's (1990) elaboration of axial and selective coding, we conceptually linked micro-level emotional states, such as acute anxiety and depressive symptoms, to macro-level factors, including lockdown mandates, institutional inaccessibility, and disrupted care pathways. Our study was further guided by a constructivist approach, as described by Bryant and Charmaz (2007), which emphasises co-constructed meaning and reflexivity. This epistemological stance was crucial for exploring the combined psychological and social effects of the pandemic on vulnerable populations, allowing us to model emotional vulnerability as context-dependent and structurally influenced. To ensure analytical rigour, we operationalised the reflexive techniques outlined by Birks and Mills (2015), whose guidance on positionality enabled us to critically assess the impact of our clinical and personal biases throughout the interpretive process of the phenomena under study. This reflexivity enhanced the validity of our findings and helped identify novel coping mechanisms, including digital peer support networks and adaptive self-regulation strategies.

Ultimately, Grounded Theory served not only as a methodological tool but also as a bridge between empirical insight and policy-relevant theory, illuminating the systemic structure of distress and resilience during pandemic crises. Furthermore, its application in pandemic settings improves public health, system preparedness, and ethical responsiveness, providing a dynamic framework for psychosocial interventions and governance in large-scale emergencies.

Integrative analysis of the population during pandemics

Understanding pandemics through the integrated lenses of ontology, epistemology, and axiology offers a multidimensional framework that significantly enriches public health discourse. Ontologically, pandemics are not merely biological disruptions but socially embedded phenomena that intersect with cultural narratives, institutional structures, and personal identities (Douglas, 2009). This perspective encourages public health to move beyond pathogen-focused models and consider how illness is experienced, narrated, and responded to within specific social contexts. Svenaeus's (2001, p. 334) notion of a disruption of one's embodied being-in-the-world highlights how public health interventions, although necessary, can exacerbate this estrangement by altering daily routines and imposing unfamiliar norms. Epistemologically, pandemic knowledge is shaped by diverse and often conflicting forms of expertise—clinical, epidemiological, and experiential—as well as by emotional and political forces such as fear, trust, and governance (Dupré and Leonelli, 2022).

Reflecting on pandemic prevention requires questioning what constitutes credible or actionable knowledge. As Lazzari and Costigliola (1993a; 1993b) observed during a pandemic, people may act against their own interests—for example, by engaging in behaviours that increase the risk of spreading a transmissible disease—despite being well-informed. This reveals a persistent gap between knowledge and behaviour, between the cognitive 'knowing what', the behavioural 'knowing how', and the emotional 'believing what'. Such a duality highlights the need to incorporate psychological, cultural, and emotional factors into models of knowledge application. Therefore, pandemic epistemology concerns not only the content of knowledge but also its creation, the trustworthiness of sources, and the decision-making processes of the population accessing information about pandemics, which is often complex, controversial, and not easily understood by laypeople.

Axiology further enriches this analysis by emphasising the role of values and ethics in shaping individual and organisational responses. Public health decisions—such as enforcing lockdowns, mandating vaccines, and distributing resources—are inherently shaped by values, reflecting ethical priorities and cultural norms (Thompson and Upshur, 2017). In the book *Water Lilies Adrift*, Lazzari, Colleoni, and Trallo (1995) examine sexually transmitted infections, particularly AIDS, as sources of moral and existential tension, in which risk perception is shaped not only by epidemiological data but also by emotional, symbolic, and identity-related factors among those at risk of contagion. Illness becomes associated with shame, desire, and self-identity, leading to behaviours such as denial, fatalism, and the eroticisation of risk—responses that challenge rationalist models of decision-making. From an axiological perspective, these behaviours reflect deeper processes of meaning-making through which individuals interpret risk in light of personal value systems.

This phenomenon explains differences in public health behaviour during pandemics—such as compliance, avoidance, and resistance—based on what individuals find meaningful, threatening, or worth sacrificing. In the book *Eros, Sexual Diseases and Society*, Lazzari, Gandolfi Colleoni, and Trallo (1996) further examine how health behaviour during widespread pandemics is shaped by cultural narratives and ethical ambivalence, showing that individuals interpret risk through interpersonal relationships and socially embedded taboos rather than solely through biomedical logic. These insights challenge traditional rationalist models and emphasise the importance of recognising the symbolic and relational aspects of health behaviour in pandemic response.

Public health and the phenomenology of risk

Phenomenological approaches to public health must examine unconscious drives and relational dynamics that shape risk behaviour, particularly when individuals act against biological self-interest to seek emotional or existential meaning. Anna Freud's concept of altruistic surrender, a form of self-sacrifice through emotional identification, offers a fundamental perspective on how individuals may internalise suffering as a meaningful act (Freud, 1936). Kaplan's (1989) interpretation of this mechanism introduces introjection, in which psychological gratification arises from internalised distress, allowing suffering to serve as a source of identity and symbolic coherence. This paradox was particularly evident during the HIV epidemic, when public health campaigns used tragic imagery to discourage unsafe practices.

For some, however, these portrayals became symbolic sanctuaries, fostering identification with suffering rather than promoting risk aversion (Kaplan, 1989). Brenner's (1988) psychology of risk studies further clarify how unconscious forces—guilt, desire, defiance—can influence behaviours that challenge rationalist models, complicating the notion that knowledge alone leads to protective action.

Lazzari and Rabottini's (2022b; 2024a) concept of Samos Syndrome captures this dynamic by describing the voluntary neglect of HIV prevention in romantic relationships between HIV-negative individuals and HIV-positive partners. This study is reported by Ceronetti (1993) and is extracted from the book *Voyage chez les lépreux* by Zambaco Pacha (1981). Their research shows how depressive states and borderline personality traits can lead to self-endangering choices, which those affected may interpret as acts of love, loyalty, or existential negotiation. In such cases, risk becomes a way of communicating: an emotionally charged means of expressing identity, attachment, and meaning. Their qualitative study of HIV-serodiscordant couples, in which one partner is HIV-positive and the other HIV-negative (Larki et al., 2020), demonstrates that these behaviours are not irrational but are deeply rooted in psychological and relational frameworks. By focusing on these dimensions, phenomenological public health can move beyond models that merely promote behavioural compliance and instead engage with the symbolic, affective, and relational aspects of risk, offering interventions that are more ethically sensitive and psychologically resonant (Table 2).

Table 2: Summative table and application in pandemics

Concept	Explanation	Application
Ontology:	Pandemics are not merely biological events but socially embedded phenomena, shaped by cultural narratives, institutions, and personal identities. Illness disrupts one's sense of normality ("unhomeliness").	Encourages public health to consider lived experiences and social contexts, not just biomedical data. Helps design interventions sensitive to the cultural and existential disruptions caused by illness and health mandates.
Epistemology:	Pandemic knowledge is shaped by clinical, epidemiological, and experiential sources and is influenced by emotions and politics. There is often a gap between knowing and acting.	Highlights the need for public health to address emotional, cultural, and psychological factors in knowledge dissemination. Supports inclusive strategies that consider how people interpret and act on information beyond rational models.
Axiology:	Values and ethics shape responses to pandemics. Risk perception is influenced by identity, emotion, and cultural norms. Illness is entangled with shame, desire, and moral tension.	Explains behavioural diversity (e.g., denial, resistance, eroticisation of risk). Supports ethically attuned public health policies that respect individual value systems and cultural narratives. Encourages moral reflection in policymaking.
Conceptualisation:	Unconscious drives (e.g., guilt, desire, defiance) influence risk-taking behaviour. Concepts such as altruistic surrender and introjection show how suffering can become meaningful or identity-forming.	Reveals why individuals may engage in self-endangering behaviours (e.g., Samos Syndrome). Helps public health understand and address emotionally charged decisions that defy rational logic. Supports psychologically informed interventions.

Concept	Explanation	Application
Behavioural Complexity:	Risk behaviour is shaped by symbolic, relational, and emotional factors—not solely by rational decision-making. People may act against self-interest for love, loyalty, or existential meaning.	Encourages public health to move beyond compliance models. Supports interventions that engage the emotional and symbolic dimensions of behaviour, particularly in vulnerable populations. Promotes empathy and relational understanding in health communication.

Conclusions

In some cases, pandemic-related health behaviours challenge the rationalist assumptions underpinning dominant public health models, particularly the belief that heightened awareness of contagion risk always leads to protective actions. This premise is fragile in pandemic contexts, where psychosocial complexities often disrupt straightforward behavioural predictions (Krieger, 2020; Bell and Green, 2022). From the perspective of pandemic epistemology, these disruptions emphasise the need for a pluralistic framework that recognises how perceptions of risk, prevention, and transmission are shaped not only by scientific modelling but also by emotional, ethical, and relational factors (Lowe et al., 2022). This complexity directly challenges rationalist models such as the Health Belief Model, revealing that perceived susceptibility and severity, as well as behavioural responses, are influenced by unconscious defences, ontological insecurity, personal biases, and early attachment experiences; these last as scaffolding in the development and internalisation of trust or mistrust in self and others (Lazzari and Masino, 2015).

Public trust in scientific authority, prevention campaigns, and the notion that public health promotion can rely on the target population's blind acceptance of rational premises may conflict with individuals' core values and their negotiation of self-reliant beliefs and communal knowledge. Preventive action, therefore, arises not only from rational deliberation but also from complex moral and relational discussions, in which the desire for intimacy and belonging can outweigh safety concerns, as illustrated by the concept of Samos Syndrome (Lazzari and Rabottini, 2024a). In this context, self-efficacy embodies ontological agency—an individual's capacity to act meaningfully in the world—which personal or temporary worldviews may hinder. Knowledge of pandemic facts alone may be insufficient to motivate the population to adopt protective behaviours, particularly among those for whom mistrust, hopelessness, or conflicting messages from the media and opinion leaders diminish belief in their ability to effect positive change (Lazzari and Masino, 2015).

Impulsivity further complicates this landscape, challenging the assumption that risk awareness leads to avoidance. While this may hold for individuals with strong self-regulatory capacities, it overlooks those whose behaviours are often shaped by unconscious conflict, sociocultural pressures, and existential distress. As Lazzari, Gandolfi Colleoni, and Trallo (1996) argue, pandemic-related behaviours are not governed solely by knowledge but by the emotional and symbolic processing of that knowledge. In this sense, impulsivity becomes an epistemological fault line—destabilising rational agency and exposing the limits of behaviourist models.

Valli and colleagues' (2002) study of youth and HIV-serodiscordant couples highlights this disruption, showing that individuals may engage in high-risk behaviours despite being fully aware of the potential consequences. These behaviours often co-occur with broader risk factors, including substance use disorders (Goedert et al., 1995), antisocial and reckless tendencies such as physical confrontations or involvement with radicalised online content (Lazzari, 2021), and impulsive actions, including occasional sexual encounters with individuals at risk of sexually transmitted diseases during emotional crises (Lazzari, Gandolfi Colleoni, and Trallo, 1996). Psychological defence mechanisms—such as denial, fantasies of invulnerability, and self-destructive relational choices—often undermine rational health behaviours and preventive measures. In psychiatric settings, persons have reported engaging in casual sexual relationships (at risk for sexually transmitted diseases) as a form of self-harm, further revealing the emotional complexity underlying pandemic-related behaviours. Consequently, the success of public health campaigns depends not only on clear communication but also on how messages are received within emotionally charged, culturally sensitive intersubjective spaces (Lazzari, Gandolfi Colleoni, and Trallo, 1996).

The aestheticisation of risk—where danger is imbued with symbolic or romanticised meaning—highlights the need for psychologically informed and culturally sensitive approaches to pandemic prevention (Lazzari, Nikolou-Walker, and Liu, 2025). These phenomena require a public health framework that incorporates epistemological nuance, ontological sensitivity, and axiological reflexivity to address the full range of human behaviour in pandemic prevention and during outbreaks.

CHAPTER 3

Ontology of Pandemics

Introduction

Lazzari and Rabottini's (2022a) study 'COVID-19, Loneliness, Social Isolation, and Risk of Dementia in Older People: A Systematic Review and Meta-Analysis' (*International Journal of Psychiatry in Clinical Practice*, 26(2), pp. 196–207) offers a comprehensive review and meta-analysis of the impact of Covid-19-related loneliness and social isolation on the risk of dementia in older adults. It combined data from longitudinal cohort studies to evaluate how social disconnection might contribute to cognitive decline.

The study found that isolated older adults, particularly during the Covid-19 lockdown, faced a significantly higher risk—up to 60%—of developing dementia, emphasising the importance of socially inclusive public health strategies during pandemic restrictions. The research presents isolation as a biologically significant condition that affects global health frameworks, vaccine uptake predictions, and ethical care planning. It also shapes interdisciplinary discussions on the ontological, epistemological, and axiological facets of pandemic vulnerability. Through this study, we regarded pandemics not merely as biological phenomena but as ontological events that fundamentally transform human identity, social meaning, and institutional coherence. Pandemics introduce what could be termed ontological layering, positioning viral outbreaks within biological systems while simultaneously permeating social structures and the existential terrains of vulnerability. Understanding pandemics ontologically requires an integrated reflection on viral dynamics, lived human suffering, and the institutional frameworks that mediate public health responses.

Dupré and Leonelli (2022), drawing on process ontology, conceptualise viruses such as SARS-CoV-2 not as static entities but as dynamic, relational processes that evolve through host interactions. This view challenges reductionist biomedical paradigms and redefines a virus (referring to those that cause pandemics) as an agent of systemic transformation rather than a discrete biological threat. Smith (2020), working within epistemic ontology, argues that the meaning of a pandemic lies not in its biological essence but in its cascading social, psychological, and moral effects. These effects manifest in phenomena such as pandemic-induced psychosis, which exemplifies ontological disruption and emphasises the need for frameworks that integrate phenomenology with relational health theory (Lazzari et al., 2020a).

Lazzari and colleagues (2020a) also document such disruptions in clinical psychiatry, where patients and practitioners alike experience altered perceptions of reality, identity, and relational meaning. These cases show that pandemics destabilise not only physical health but also the ontological foundations of human experience. Ultimately, this reflection treats pandemics as ontological dislocations, epistemological challenges, and axiological dilemmas—events that demand ethically sensitive and conceptually rigorous responses. Therefore, pandemics are not merely viral episodes but profound social and existential ruptures. As Lazzari and colleagues (2020b) note, Covid-19 fractured core aspects of human life: it reshaped meaning, changed relationships, and fragmented identity. Clinical practice itself became a space of ontological uncertainty, where caregivers and patients navigated fear, isolation, and the breakdown of familiar norms. These disruptions call for a conceptual shift, one that recognises pandemics as crises of being, knowing, and valuing and seeks to understand the lived experience of those affected.

A 2020 case report published in the journal *Psychiatria Danubina* describes the psychiatric effects of the Covid-19 pandemic, focusing on the first admission of a 50-year-old man who tested negative for Covid-19 but exhibited acute paranoid delusions (Lazzari et al., 2020b). He believed impostors had replaced his family members and that the virus was a government-engineered tool for population control. Motivated by these beliefs, he planned to commit suicide, viewing it as a protective act against further psychological and physical suffering (Lazzari et al., 2020b). Diagnosed with reactive psychosis and an acute paranoid reaction, he responded to antipsychotic medication and was discharged within a week (Lazzari et al., 2020b).

This case illustrates how pandemic-induced existential fear can lead to ontological disintegration—an erosion of perceptions of reality, identity, and relational meaning. It also emphasises that any pandemic is not merely a biological threat but a deep ontological force that disrupts how individuals experience their being-in-the-world. Building on this, Guerrero Fernandez (2022) introduces the concept of ontological stratification, arguing that pandemics must be understood across multiple, intersecting layers of reality, including biological, social, and existential. These layers are shaped by contingency and vulnerability, revealing how viral outbreaks infiltrate not only the body but also the symbolic and relational fabric of human life.

Ontological stratification offers a framework for understanding the pandemic as a complex, multidimensional event that disrupts normative structures and exposes the fragility of systems that produce meaning. Together, these perspectives foster a conceptual shift in public health discourse, recognising a pandemic as a crisis of existence rather than merely an infection.

Pandemic ontology resists simple definitions; instead, it comprises a network of conditions that shape human life across biological, social, and existential dimensions. To understand pandemics ontologically, we must move beyond reductionist models that focus solely on viral behaviour in laboratory settings or on clinical data. A broader reflection is needed, one that considers how viral biology, lived suffering, and institutional systems interact to produce crises not only in biological laboratories but also in homes, bodies, and the symbolic frameworks through which individuals create meaning and manage uncertainty.

We could strengthen our unified theories and recommendations for pandemics by building on previous research into psychosocial responses to infectious diseases, including the AIDS epidemic, which showed that even well-informed individuals may ignore public health advice despite understanding the risks to themselves and others (Lazzari, Colleoni, and Trallo, 1995). Such behaviour highlights a significant tension between traditional notions of rationality—usually defined by clarity of thought and logical reasoning—and the irrational reactions that can arise under psychological and pandemic anxiety.

Standard definitions of rationality, such as those from the Cambridge Dictionary (2024b), describe it as "the quality of being based on clear thought and reason, or of making decisions based on clear thought and reason." This view emphasises cognitive coherence and diminishes the role of emotion, instinct, and social meaning in shaping human behaviour and thoughts. However, as pandemic circumstances demonstrate, decisions are rarely made in isolation from emotional and relational influences. The gap between normative rationality and actual behaviour shows that public health compliance is not merely about conveying knowledge but about ontological stability. When fear, isolation, and existential threats dominate, individuals may act in ways that contradict instrumental logic, not because they lack understanding but because their sense of self, agency, and relational coherence has been destabilised. Pandemic ontology, therefore, must recognise these complex realities, acknowledging that health behaviour is influenced as much by meaning-making and vulnerability as by information and reason.

The concept of irrationalism has long stood in contrast to formal models of rationality, particularly during periods of psychological stress and existential threat. Traditional accounts of rational behaviour emphasise clarity of thought, logical consistency, and reason-based decision-making. Yet these models often overlook more profound influences—emotion, instinct, and cultural values—that shape what is generally regarded as "reasonable" behaviour. As Lazzari and Masino (2015) argue in their exploration of health psychology and philosophy, human responses to crises are rarely driven solely by logic; instead, they reflect complex emotional and existential forces that challenge standard assumptions about rationality. This tension becomes particularly evident in public health emergencies, where individual and collective decisions often defy instrumental logic.

According to the Cambridge Dictionary (2024a), irrationality is defined as "not using reason or clear thinking," a definition that supports a behavioural interpretation centred on cognitive deviation. However, this framing oversimplifies the broader conceptual discourse. The Collins English Dictionary (2024) describes irrationalism as "a theory that nonrational forces govern the universe," while Dictionary.com (2024) expands it to "an attitude or belief based on nonrational grounds." These definitions indicate that irrationalism is not merely a cognitive error but a worldview that questions the dominance of reason and recognises the roles of emotion, intuition, and existential perspective in shaping human behaviour.

Professor Borlotti (2015) elaborates on this by identifying key traits associated with irrational behaviour: impulsivity, lack of self-awareness, failure to comprehend complexity, and excessive pride. These traits are not random deviations but patterned responses to uncertainty and threat. Drawing on Plato's *Republic*, Borlotti (2015) notes that the soul comprises three elements—reason, which seeks truth; spirit, which craves dignity and recognition; and appetite, which pursues pleasure and self-interest. When appetite and spirit override reason, behaviour shifts from deliberation to emotional survival. In this light, irrationalism is not a flaw but an adaptive strategy for navigating crises when conventional rationality proves insufficient. During pandemics, such non-rational responses reveal how meaning-making, identity, and ethical orientation are reconfigured under pressure, demanding a more nuanced understanding of human agency.

When individuals prioritise basic desires—such as pleasure, dominance, or emotional fulfilment—over reason and honour, their behaviour often shifts from principled reflection to impulsive, self-interested action. As Borlotti (2015) explains, this shift signifies a move away from traditional rationality and the rise of irrationalism as an epistemic alternative. Rather than viewing irrationalism as a cognitive flaw, Borlotti (2015) describes it as a response grounded in emotion, existential perspective, and adaptive survival strategies. This reinterpretation is particularly relevant during public emergencies and pandemics, when psychological stress and existential threats undermine normative reasoning. In such contexts, non-rational reactions reveal how human meaning-making resists simple explanations and instead reflects deeper ontological and emotional processes.

Standard definitions of rationality, such as those from the Cambridge Dictionary (2024b), emphasise "clear thinking" and logical decision-making. However, this view overlooks the complexity of real-world behaviour, particularly under pressure. Irrationalism, far from being synonymous with chaos, reflects the mental and existential strategies individuals employ when logic alone cannot explain their experience. During pandemic outbreaks, many people experience a reversal of rational balance; fear, uncertainty, and emotional overload override cautious thought. This disorientation can hinder adaptive self-preservation and distort the pursuit of well-being, as shown in earlier clinical research on AIDS-related behavioural patterns (Lazzari et al., 1994) and in more recent studies on borderline personality disorder and pandemic susceptibility (Lazzari et al., 2025).

Clinical observations during Covid-19 further demonstrate that isolation and extended societal restrictions can heighten emotional distress and reinforce fundamental beliefs, such as solipsism, the idea that only one's own mind and interpretation of truth reliably exist. A solipsistic worldview, as defined by Merriam-Webster (2024) and Encyclopaedia Britannica (2024b), undermines both collective responsibility and mutual recognition, both of which are essential for effective public health engagement. During pandemics, solipsistic tendencies may manifest as withdrawal, denialism, or refusal to engage with shared norms and truths, emphasising the need for public health strategies that address not only informational gaps but also existential and solipsistic interpretations of biological realities.

Research rationale and conceptual framing

The Covid-19 pandemic exposed notable vulnerabilities in older people, not only in their biological susceptibility to infection but also in their cognitive and psychosocial resilience. Our study (Lazzari and Rabottini, 2022a) examines how pandemic-related social isolation and loneliness, two intense psychosocial stressors, contribute to neurocognitive decline and social deterioration. Through a systematic review and meta-analysis of longitudinal cohort studies, the research integrates epidemiological data with public mental health priorities, providing a comprehensive evidence base to guide intervention strategies and policy development (Lazzari and Rabottini, 2022a).

Our conceptual framework extends beyond pathogen-focused models by defining isolation as a condition shaped by structural and social factors and with enduring cognitive effects. It promotes a biopsychosocial approach to understanding vulnerability during pandemics. Our research, therefore, seeks to assess the risk of dementia associated with social disconnection in pandemic contexts. A key methodological advance was to harmonise the accuracy of meta-analysis with the complexity of psychosocial concepts such as loneliness and relational deprivation. Through iterative coding and stratified sensitivity analysis, our research examined how behavioural and structural factors—such as living arrangements, access to care, and emotional coping—interact with vulnerability during lockdowns. This approach provided more profound insight into the mechanisms linking isolation to cognitive decline, thereby strengthening both the technical rigour and conceptual clarity of pandemic-related mental health research.

Policy and pandemic preparedness

The findings from Lazzari and Rabottini (2022a) align with global and national public health guidelines, particularly those issued by the WHO (World Health Organization, 2020) and the NHS (National Health Service England, 2023), which advocate socially inclusive care strategies during health emergencies. By demonstrating the link between enforced isolation and accelerated cognitive decline in older adults, our study contributes to vital debates on ethical triage and resource allocation in long-term care settings. It shows that frail individuals, already lacking sufficient social and emotional support, face heightened risks when subjected to lockdown measures. These insights emphasise the importance of integrating cognitive dignity into emergency planning, ensuring that older adults (and other vulnerable groups, such as those with limited autonomy, very ill individuals, or those with long-term physical and mental health conditions) are not only protected from infection but also supported in maintaining mental and relational well-being. Our study thus advocates a shift in pandemic preparedness from reactive containment to proactive, ethically grounded care models that prioritise neurocognitive resilience and social connectedness among vulnerable groups.

Conceptual extensions of pandemic research

Our research (Lazzari and Rabottini, 2022a) has established a key reference point in the interdisciplinary study of pandemics, particularly by emphasising the cognitive risks older adults face during enforced social isolation. By demonstrating the neurocognitive consequences of loneliness and disconnection, our work suggests a broader rethinking of how isolation is conceptualised across multiple disciplines.

Ontologically, our study redefines social isolation as a biologically significant state rather than merely a social experience. Axially, it emphasises the moral obligation to protect cognitive dignity and relational well-being among vulnerable groups, urging public health systems to embed values of inclusion and care within pandemic emergency responses. Epistemologically, our findings show how knowledge of isolation is developed, validated, and utilised, encouraging scholars to consider emotional, cultural, and structural factors in models of risk and prevention. As a result, our research has been cited by other scholars, influencing both theoretical frameworks and practical strategies in pandemic preparedness and geriatric mental health.

Ontological impact: Reframing isolation as a neurocognitive condition

Pandemics are ontological disruptions that reshape identity, rationality, and meaning across biological, social, and existential dimensions. They challenge fixed models of health and reasoning, demanding integrated, ethically mindful responses. Pandemics do more than disrupt biological systems; they fracture identities and add ontological layers by situating viral outbreaks within social frameworks and existential vulnerabilities. Understanding pandemics ontologically entails analysing viral dynamics, lived suffering, and institutional responses.

Smith's epistemic ontology holds that the meaning of a pandemic arises not from its inherent nature but from its effects—social, psychological, and moral (Smith, 2019). Cases of pandemic-induced psychosis, such as Lazzari and colleagues (2020a; 2020b; 2020c; 2020d), describe a man's delusional response to Covid-19, illustrating ontological disintegration—a breakdown in the perception of reality, identity, and relational meaning (Jukić et al., 2020). Guerrero Fernandez (2022) extends this idea through ontological stratification, suggesting that pandemics operate across layered realities—biological, social, and existential—where contingency and vulnerability intersect. Lazzari and colleagues (2020d) note that Covid-19 fractured core aspects of human life, reshaping meaning, transforming relationships, and fragmenting identity. Clinical practice became a domain of ontological uncertainty, with caregivers and patients navigating fear, isolation, and the erosion of familiar norms. These disruptions demonstrate that pandemics are not merely viral events but existential crises that challenge individuals' experience of being-in-the-world.

We have already established that ontological instability during crises disrupts rational decision-making. Prior research (Lazzari et al., 2021) shows that even well-informed individuals may disregard public health guidance under psychological stress. While traditional definitions of rationality (Cambridge Dictionary, 2024b) emphasise clarity and reason, they overlook the influence of emotion, instinct, and sociocultural factors. Irrationalism, often defined as the absence of reason (Cambridge Dictionary, 2024a), is reinterpreted as an epistemic stance shaped by emotional and existential elements. Philosophical perspectives—from Borlotti's (2015) discussion of impulsivity and pride to Plato's tripartite soul (Plato, trans. 2007)—demonstrate how non-rational forces can override reflective judgement. In pandemic contexts, irrationalism serves as a strategic response to uncertainty, supported by broader definitions from sources such as Collins and Dictionary.com.

During pandemics, emotional disorientation can impair self-preservation and distort well-being. Isolation may reawaken solipsistic beliefs—the idea that only one's own mind is sure to exist—thereby undermining collective responsibility and mutual recognition (Lazzari and Rabottini, 2024a). We define irrational health behaviour as any action that increases an individual's risk of infection despite awareness of the consequences. This process aligns with medical capacity assessments, which evaluate understanding, retention, reasoning, and communication of the information provided, and the weighing of pros and cons of one's own decisions linked to that information (e.g., risks and benefits of not wearing a mask during pandemic outbreaks) (GMC, 2024). Disruptions in these domains can undermine decision-making (GMC, 2024) and hinder pandemic prevention efforts.

Guarnera, Yuen, and Macpherson (2023) cite our study in their narrative review of cognitive ageing, using it to frame the neurocognitive consequences of social disconnection. Their work reinforces the ontological shift proposed in our research: that isolation, especially during pandemics, is not merely a social or emotional experience but a biologically significant condition with measurable effects on brain health. Barton, Lee, and Cacioppo (2023) extend this perspective by integrating our findings into a translational neuroscience model, identifying loneliness as a neurobiological risk factor for dementia and incorporating it into predictive frameworks for cognitive decline. Similarly, Corbett and colleagues (2022) draw directly on our longitudinal data to demonstrate notable cognitive deterioration in older adults during and after the Covid-19 pandemic, further supporting our proposition that isolation acts as a progressive and degenerative force. Together, these citations affirm the ontological reality of isolation as a condition with structural, emotional, and neurobiological dimensions, positioning our work as a foundational reference in the ongoing discourse on ageing, vulnerability, and pandemic-related cognitive risk.

Axiological contributions: Reassessing values in healthcare

Our research has prompted a rethinking of pandemics across three key phenomenological dimensions: (1) ontologically, it redefines isolation as a biologically embedded and cognitively meaningful state rather than merely a social inconvenience; (2) epistemologically, it alters how isolation is measured, modelled, and understood across disciplines, incorporating emotional, structural, and behavioural aspects; and (3) axiologically, it emphasises the ethical responsibility to promote connection, care, and dignity within health systems and emerging technologies especially during pandemics.

Rather than merely serving as a passive citation, our work has evolved into a conceptual framework—a lens through which the pandemic's most significant human impacts are being reinterpreted, reframed, and operationalised across clinical, technological, and public health fields. The first ten peer-reviewed studies citing Lazzari and Rabottini (2022a) highlight its interdisciplinary influence across neuroscience, public health, behavioural science, and geriatric care. These citations demonstrate that our research has become a conceptual and methodological bridge for emerging studies on pandemic vulnerability, cognitive ageing, and social determinants of health.

Neurocognitive and Ontological Impact: Guarnera, Yuen, and Macpherson (2023) cite our work to contextualise the neurocognitive effects of social disconnection in ageing, thereby reinforcing our ontological framing of isolation as a biologically significant condition. Barton, Lee, and Cacioppo (2024) incorporate our findings into a translational neuroscience model, positioning loneliness as a neurobiological risk factor for dementia. Corbett and colleagues (2022) use our longitudinal data to demonstrate cognitive decline among older adults during and after the Covid-19 pandemic.

Epistemological Influence and Global Adaptation: Prommas, Chen, and Lin (2023) extend our analytical framework to evaluate global health outcomes, demonstrating its flexibility across diverse cultural contexts. Luchetti, Sutin, and Terracciano (2022) cite our study in the largest meta-analysis to date on loneliness and dementia risk, thereby improving measurement criteria for cognitive decline. Liu, Zhang, and Wang (2023) utilise our framework to link sensory impairments to isolation and dementia risk among middle-aged and older adults in China, illustrating its effectiveness in both cross-sectional and longitudinal studies.

Axiological Reach and Ethical Reframing: Hanna, Smith, and Thomas (2023) cite our findings to link social isolation to dietary decline, suggesting that nutritional well-being is closely tied to relational bonds. Kang, Yamamoto, and Saito (2023) utilise our research to examine the role of care robots in elder care, raising ethical questions about technology-mediated empathy and the value of human interaction. Pronk and colleagues (2025) cite our study to contextualise social determinants of health within an ecological model, emphasising the importance of relational integrity and community-based care in population health science. Alam, Choudhury, and Rahman (2023) incorporate our findings into behavioural forecasting models, treating social isolation as a variable influencing vaccine uptake.

Impact Summary: Collectively, these citations demonstrate how Lazzari and Rabottini (2022a) have catalysed a rethinking of pandemics across three phenomenological dimensions:

- *Ontologically,* it redefines isolation as a biologically embedded and cognitively consequential condition.
- *Epistemologically,* it reshapes how isolation is measured, modelled, and understood across disciplines.
- *Axiologically,* it elevates the moral imperative of connection, care, and dignity in health systems and technologies.

Ontological disruption across population layers during pandemics

Pandemics disrupt the fundamental aspects of human life across all age groups, not just among older adults. The disruption of daily routines, social connections, and embodied freedoms fractures individuals' sense of continuity, identity, and embeddedness in the world. For children, this rupture may cause developmental disorientation and weaken the process of meaning-making through play. Adolescents experience identity diffusion and epistemic confusion as key transitions are interrupted. Working-age adults face existential insecurity due to economic instability, job loss, and a breakdown in future planning. Even those not directly affected by the illness may suffer ontological shock triggered by media saturation, symbolic contagion, and anticipatory grief (Lazzari and Rabottini, 2025a; 2025b). This is not merely a psychological disturbance; it indicates a deeper reconfiguration of how individuals see themselves as agents, knowers, and moral subjects. Drawing on earlier publications, this framework considers pandemic-induced ontological instability as a trans-stratal phenomenon that undermines cognitive integrity, ethical orientation, and epistemic trust. It calls for a rethinking of mental health interventions that go beyond simply managing symptoms to restoring ontological coherence through relational scaffolding, narrative repair, and ethically conscious care.

Previous research on sexually transmitted diseases (Lazzari and Costigliola, 1993a; 1993b; Lazzari, Gandolfi Colleoni, and Trallo, 1996) demonstrated that symbolic contagion and existential fear influence interpersonal dynamics and moral reasoning—insights that remain highly relevant amid pandemic-related disruptions. In social sciences, ontology serves as the fundamental lens through which researchers understand the nature and structure of social reality. It involves questioning whether institutions, norms, roles, and relationships exist independently of human perception or are constructed through interaction and discourse. The ontological stance adopted by a researcher determines which phenomena are regarded as legitimate subjects of inquiry and influences assumptions about their permanence, measurability, and relationships within broader societal systems. Key ontological questions include: What makes a social phenomenon real? Is reality objectively fixed or subjectively experienced? Does it remain static, or is it continually reshaped through social practice and language (Grix, 2010)?

In this context, pandemics act as ontological disruptors, fragmenting the lived realities and identities of individuals and communities. They challenge assumptions about stability, agency, and relational embeddedness by dismantling routines, roles, and symbolic structures. Our studies have shown that in the face of deadly diseases, people often reinterpret life's meaning and existential outlook; this ontological recalibration influences how they perceive themselves and others. Epistemologically, pandemics reduce trust in knowledge systems, exposing tensions between scientific authority, public belief, and the spread of misinformation (Lazzari and Costigliola, 1993a; 1993b). Methodologically, these conditions call for adaptable, ethically sensitive research designs, particularly in healthcare, where isolation, trauma, and structural inequalities challenge traditional methods and require context-aware inquiry. This triadic disruption—ontological, epistemological, and methodological—calls for a rethinking of how the social sciences engage with crisis, vulnerability, and the evolving contours of human experience.

As already seen, drawing on the principles of process ontology, Dupré and Leonelli (2022) reconceptualise viruses such as SARS-CoV-2 not as fixed, isolated entities but as dynamic and relational processes. In their view, viral behaviour is not intrinsic to the virus alone but emerges through its interactions with hosts and environments. This challenges conventional biomedical models that treat viruses as static biological threats, instead emphasising their fluid, context-sensitive nature. Pandemics, therefore, are not merely events caused by a pathogen. Instead, they are ontological disruptors that reshape how individuals experience existence, embodiment, and relational meaning. This disruption is vividly illustrated in cases of pandemic-induced psychosis, such as the euthanasia attempt to escape the Covid-19 threat reported in the journal *Psychiatria Danubina* (Lazzari et al., 2020b), where existential fear fractured the individual's sense of identity, reality, and moral orientation. Such episodes demonstrate the profound psychological and ontological consequences of pandemics, which extend beyond physical illness to destabilise the very foundations of selfhood and social embeddedness. Building on Smith's (2020) epistemic ontology, this framework argues that the real impact of a pandemic lies not in its biological properties but in its social, psychological, and moral reverberations.

The experience of psychosis during a pandemic demonstrates an ontological rupture, a breakdown in the coherence of being that necessitates integrative approaches to care. These approaches must blend phenomenological insight with relational health theory, as recommended by de Lima (2020) and Rittmannsberger and colleagues (2022), to address the existential aspects of suffering. Pandemics, therefore, are not merely biomedical events; they are transformative social phenomena that displace meaning, rupture relationships, and fracture identity, as Lazzari and colleagues (2020a) have shown. Pandemic outbreaks destabilise fundamental aspects of human life, transforming clinical environments into spaces of ontological uncertainty characterised by fear, isolation, and the collapse of normative structures (Lazzari et al., 2020a; 2020b). This necessitates a reorientation of mental healthcare toward ethically sensitive, relational interventions that re-establish ontological coherence and address the full range of human vulnerability during times of crisis.

Guerrero Fernandez (2022) introduces ontological stratification to frame pandemics as layered phenomena—biological, social, and existential—that converge through contingency and vulnerability. This multidimensional approach challenges reductionist models by urging scholars to consider how viral biology, human suffering, and institutional systems co-produce crises in lived spaces such as bodies, homes, and symbolic environments. It emphasises that pandemics are not solely biomedical events but complex disruptions unfolding across multiple strata of human experience. Empirical studies, such as Nie, Zhang, and Li (2021), reveal that individuals may ignore public health guidance even when fully aware of the risks, exposing a disconnect between normative rationality—defined as decision-making based on clear, logical thought (Cambridge Dictionary, 2025b)—and the emotionally driven, socially embedded behaviours that emerge under stress. In response, Lazzari and Rabottini (2025a; 2025b) argue for public health strategies that combine epidemiological data with psychosocial insight and phenomenological depth. Such integration is vital for addressing real-world issues of compliance, resilience, and ethical complexity.

Within this conceptual landscape, our quadruplex helix of pandemic health ontology offers a framework for understanding how solipsism, irrationalism, and evolving ideas of self and others shape responses to health communication and containment strategies (Lazzari and Rabottini, 2025a; 2025b). The model describes how social layers—individuals, dyads, peer groups, and cultural communities—generate diverse interpretive and behavioural patterns, often misaligned with public health rationality (Lazzari and Rabottini, 2025a; 2025b).

- *Micro level:* The solitary individual operates from a belief system rooted in subjective certainty and solipsism: "What I believe is true; any contradiction must be false." This epistemic rigidity fosters resistance to protective measures such as mask-wearing or vaccination, not because of a lack of information, but because such interventions are perceived as threats to autonomy and invulnerability.

- *Meso level:* Within dyadic relationships, health beliefs are influenced by emotional intimacy. Shared convictions may evolve into mutually reinforced biased narratives, as seen in *folie à deux*, where one partner often assumes interpretive dominance, shaping perceptions of risk and appropriate action.
- *Macro level:* Peer groups shape identity through oppositional logic. Health beliefs serve as symbolic markers of belonging: "What we believe may conflict with dominant norms, but it defines who we are." This often leads to selective adherence to or rejection of public health advice, driven by the need to maintain group cohesion and ideological uniqueness (Lazzari, Costley, and Nikolou-Walker, 2024).
- *Mega level:* At the mega level, beliefs and behaviours about pandemics are shaped by national identity, political culture, and institutional narratives. A country's view of what constitutes a pandemic and how it should be handled reflects its broader ontological and ideological commitments, whether as a biopolitical emergency, a moral test of solidarity, or a defence of personal freedom. Symbolic resources, including national myths, media discourse, and policy frameworks, shape public health responses. This level shows how state-led narratives shape collective behaviour, often producing competing interpretations and fragmented compliance. The mega level thus presents pandemics as nationalised phenomena in which biology, politics, and meaning-making converge.

These stratified dynamics echo earlier ideas about health and meaning-making (Lazzari and Masino, 2015). They are further elaborated in our psychosocial and public health framework (Lazzari and Rabottini, 2025a; 2025b), which examines how existential vulnerability, symbolic identity, and moral reasoning shape pandemic-related behaviours across diverse populations. The quadruplex helix thus offers a comprehensive perspective on the ontological, epistemological, and axiological dimensions of pandemic responses, providing a pathway towards more ethically attentive and socially responsive public health strategies. We argue that solipsistic worldviews—where individuals believe only their own minds are certain—can undermine collective responsibility and hinder mutual recognition, both of which are essential for practical public health efforts.

In pandemic contexts, such worldviews encourage behavioural resistance, especially when public health measures are viewed as threats to personal autonomy rather than shared ethical obligations. We define irrational health behaviour during a pandemic as any action that elevates individuals' personal risk of contracting or transmitting an infectious disease, even when they possess adequate knowledge of the illness, its consequences, and transmission methods. This aligns with principles of capacity assessment in clinical medicine, which evaluate whether a person can understand relevant risks (cognitive aspect), retain information sufficiently to act upon it, weigh the benefits and drawbacks of decisions, and communicate their choices to others, such as healthcare providers (NHS, 2024). Any disruption in these stages—whether caused by emotional distress, cognitive overload, or existential disorientation—can result in diminished capacity and decreased prevention, as evidenced by prior research on sexually transmitted infections and AIDS-related behaviours (Lazzari, 1992).

Moreover, solipsism highlights a significant gap between propositional knowledge ('knowing what'), practical knowledge ('knowing how'), and lived conviction ('believing what'), which often leads to resistance to prevention campaigns. Individuals may intellectually understand the rationale for public health measures but emotionally or existentially reject them, especially when these measures clash with their internal sense of reality, autonomy, or control. To interpret these behaviours, the ontological turn in philosophy offers a helpful perspective. It encourages us to view pandemic health behaviours through the lens of irrationalism—a metaphysical tradition that emphasises intuition, emotion, and volition over reason. As Encyclopaedia Britannica (2024a) notes, irrationalism is not merely a deviation from logic but a worldview that questions the primacy of rationality itself. In this context, irrational health behaviour becomes an adaptive response to uncertainty and threat, shaped by existential vulnerability rather than cognitive failure. Recognising this complexity is vital for designing public health strategies that address not only the intellect but also the emotional and ontological aspects of human experience.

The quadruplex helix illustrates that pandemic health behaviour is not merely a matter of individual choice or mental capacity. Instead, it is rooted in layered social structures—personal, relational, communal, and national—that shape how people interpret, follow, or resist advice. This perspective aligns with existing models of teamwork and professional interactions in healthcare, where handovers and collaboration are shaped by shared beliefs, identities, and relational understandings (Lazzari, Costley, and Nikolou-Walker, 2024).

Table 3: Quadruplex helix of pandemic health ontology

Level	Social Unit	Core Belief Dynamics	Behavioural Implications
Micro Level:	Individual	Subjective certainty (solipsism): "What I believe is true; any contradiction must be false."	Rejection of protective measures (e.g., masks, vaccines) is not due to ignorance but to a perceived threat to cognitive autonomy and control.
Meso Level:	Dyadic Couple	Shared belief systems reinforced through emotional intimacy; potential for *folie à deux*.	Health narratives are mutually sustained; one partner may dominate the framing of risk and truth.
Macro Level:	Peer Group	Identity shaped through opposition; health beliefs as symbols of belonging.	Selective adherence or rejection of public health logic to maintain group cohesion and ideological distinctiveness.
Cultural & Community Level:	Cultural & Collectives	Interpretive traditions and collective memory influence health behaviour at scale.	Community-wide responses are shaped by historical mistrust, symbolic resistance, and cultural narratives.

Ontological anchors and the disjunction of knowledge and conviction

Psychology has long debated the conflict between rational knowledge and lived belief. At the core of this debate lies an ontological foundation, the fundamental perspective through which individuals perceive reality. When this foundation shifts towards solipsism and irrationalism, the self becomes the sole arbiter of truth, and the immediacy of intuition, will, and emotion replaces reason's authority.

This orientation creates a notable divide between propositional knowledge and lived conviction. Understanding what is true in theory—through science, logic, or public debate—does not ensure that one will believe it in practice. Rational statements, no matter how carefully constructed, often fail to reach the level of conviction, which is more influenced by emotional resonance than by logical argument. In such a framework, knowledge is recognised but not internalised; truth is acknowledged but not genuinely felt.

The implications of this disjunction are evident in public health behaviours during pandemics. Campaigns to prevent harm and promote well-being rely on the persuasive power of evidence, statistics, and logical arguments. However, when individuals interpret these messages through a solipsistic lens, they do not perceive them as universal truths but as external impositions. This leads to resistance to prevention campaigns, not out of ignorance but because of differing interpretations. Public health messages, grounded in rational universality, clash with personal belief sovereignty, creating a divide between collective reason and individual conviction.

Thus, the philosophical issue is not only epistemological but also existential. When linked to irrationalism, the foundation of ontology resists the influence of shared rationality and redefines truth as a matter of subjective immediacy. In this conflict, the universality of reason confronts the sovereignty of belief, and the emphasis on personal interpretation challenges the possibility of collective consensus. The story of resistance is therefore not accidental but innate: it emerges from how individuals establish their reality and cognitive or behavioural priorities, favouring lived conviction over propositional knowledge.

Resistance to public health guidance—such as viewing mask-wearing to avoid contagion as a sign of weakness—often stems more from social performance concerns than from scientific evidence. In these cases, adherence to or defiance of health norms is driven by a desire for peer validation and social acceptance. At both macro and micro levels of the quadruplex helix, collective cultural beliefs take precedence. Narratives such as "Our nation is immune" or "Illness is foreign or immoral" encourage politicised behaviour, often fuelled by distrust of international health organisations and exacerbated by misinformation. This cultural exceptionalism hinders the adoption of preventive behaviours, especially when illness is portrayed as an external threat rather than a shared human experience. As Lazzari and colleagues (2020a; 2020b; 2020c) observe in early psychiatric case reports during Covid-19, such resistance is not solely cognitive but also deeply relational and symbolic, rooted in social belief systems that can either support or oppose public health efforts.

The quadruplex helix framework situates pandemic behaviour within the scope of conceptual and phenomenological exploration, illustrating how disruptions in public health compliance reflect deep ontological tensions. By engaging affective epistemologies and the subtle links between self and others, it expands the concept of prevention beyond solely rationalist approaches. Pandemic responses are not merely statistical figures; they are experienced, emotionally charged phenomena. Critical moments such as lockdowns, diagnostic tests, and witnessing illness expose the delicate ontological foundations of life and the intricate ethical dimensions of decision-making. Risk becomes embodied and rooted in existence as individuals navigate vulnerability, relational exposure, and uncertainty (Lazzari et al., 2021). Viewing pandemic behaviours through this perspective, they embody human meaning-making amid ontological upheaval. Accidents (e.g., accidental contagion)—whether tragic, predictable, or random—rarely lack meaning in public perception. Instead, they might reveal patterns of choice, neglect, and unconscious intention.

Resistance to protective measures during Covid-19 cannot be fully explained by ignorance or negligence. Instead, it reveals a more profound ambivalence in how people negotiate bodily boundaries, interpersonal exposure, and their existential position in a destabilised world. Risk-taking reflects internal conflict, with the pursuit of gratification clashing with the instinct for self-preservation. Among populations vulnerable to sexually transmitted infections, this tension is evident in oscillations between libidinal urgency and avoidance, impulsive surrender, and unconscious awareness of danger (Lazzari and Costigliola, 1993a). These choices often bypass reflective reasoning, operating through preconscious mechanisms that elude traditional public health models (Lazzari et al., 1991).

To interpret these behaviours, we adopt a phenomenological perspective, drawing on the concept of Samos Syndrome, a form of pathophilia, defined as an unconscious attraction to illness. First introduced at psychiatric congresses and later elaborated in the clinical literature, Samos Syndrome treats health-risking behaviours as symbolic acts that reflect internal conflicts rather than signs of unawareness (Lazzari, 2012). Our ethnographic research emphasises that individuals with pathological personality traits may engage in illness-seeking behaviours as a means of self-punishment, fulfilment, escape, or attachment. These dynamics challenge the adequacy of rationalist models of behavioural prevention and highlight the importance of understanding how existential vulnerability shapes health choices during pandemics.

Conclusions

We argue that pandemics are ontological crises, that is, disruptions that undermine bodily autonomy, relational intimacy, and the flow of everyday time. Vulnerability, expressed through breath, touch, and proximity, blurs the perceived boundary between self and other, transforming the body into a site of existential exposure. Rejecting preventive measures such as mask-wearing or social distancing during pandemics may not simply stem from ignorance or defiance. It can be understood as an existential act of protest, a denial of mortality and of the tension between Eros and Thanatos, intimacy and withdrawal, vitality and surrender (Wikipedia Contributors, 2023). Martin and colleagues (2022) view the pandemic not merely as a biomedical event but as a profound human experience that necessitates compassion, narrative understanding, and a renewed philosophy of care.

During pandemics such as HIV/AIDS and Covid-19, what appears accidental often reveals deeper psychological and ontological vulnerabilities. Lazzari and Rabottini (2024a) describe how critical incidents—seemingly random or preventable events—carry symbolic significance, particularly when individuals engage in high-risk behaviours, such as unprotected sex with casual partners, that place them at risk of sexually transmissible diseases. The World Health Organization (WHO, 2025) characterises critical incidents as emotionally destabilising, unexpected events that go beyond normal experience. Although behaviours such as ignoring distancing protocols are preventable from an epidemiological perspective (WHO, 2023), they often occur amid missed signals, delayed decisions, and internal struggles. As demonstrated during the early AIDS crisis, some individuals might engage in risky activities despite clear public health warnings during pandemic outbreaks. These incidents, while often survivable with adequate support, can overwhelm coping mechanisms and expose unconscious ambivalence.

Freud (1901) and Brenner (1988) offer psychological insights into how seemingly reckless actions may mask deeper motives, including self-harm, fatalism, or existential expression. Brenner's interpretation of Freud's *The Psychopathology of Everyday Life* suggests that accidents can reveal unconscious motives—such as punishment, atonement, or self-sacrifice—rather than being simple mistakes. This framework helps explain pandemic-related risk behaviours, in which individuals knowingly engage in unsafe practices, thereby exposing the tension between immediate gratification and psychological vulnerability (Lazzari, cited in AdoleScienza.it, 2025). Lazzari and Costigliola (1993a; 1993b) observed that such behaviours often bypass rational deterrents and are driven by unresolved psychological conflicts. In some cases, the threat of contagion becomes a means of self-harm or symbolic fulfilment.

Mass media further reinforced these patterns by portraying marginalised individuals receiving care, a dynamic Kaplan (1989) termed altruistic surrender, in which personal gratification is sacrificed to meet others' needs, leading to satisfaction through introjection. During the AIDS epidemic, this phenomenon was particularly evident in cases of Samos Syndrome, where HIV-negative persons in stable relationships with HIV-positive partners intentionally engaged in unprotected sexual relations, as an act of existential commitment or sacrificial love (Lazzari, cited in Psicologi Italia, 2025). Lazzari and colleagues (2020a; 2020b; 2020c; 2020d) regarded these actions not as impulsive but as conceptually driven choices; gestures of emotional depth and relational transcendence.

These decisions are underpinned by complex psychological narratives centred on redemption, devotion, and a longing for unconditional love. For some, intimacy becomes more meaningful not despite the risk of contagion and casualties, but because of them. The closeness forged in these moments carries emotional significance that transcends typical boundaries (Lazzari, 1992). Durkheim's (1991) concept of altruistic self-sacrifice helps frame these behaviours as internally motivated acts of service to a perceived greater cause, rather than externally imposed obligations. In this context, pandemic behaviours not only reflect epidemiological trends but also serve as attempts to make sense of life, challenging the adequacy of rationalist models and advocating for psychologically sensitive public health strategies.

Social isolation during pandemics significantly impairs cognitive, social, and interpersonal functions, undermining individual well-being and fragmenting collective understanding. Socially, isolation during pandemics erodes trust, damages relational networks, and hampers shared meaning-making, leading to confusion about knowledge and disengagement from public health messages. Interpersonally, the absence of early supportive caregiving (from early life) causes emotional instability, identity issues, and morally complex decisions, particularly during vulnerable developmental stages. These elements affect trust in others and in one's own choices. These disruptions give rise to complex belief systems—ranging from personal absolutism to ideologically reinforced narratives within peer groups and cultural communities—resulting in diverse perspectives on risk, truth, and authority. Compliance with health measures depends more on relational context, emotional bonds, and symbolic belonging than on access to information alone. Recognising these ontological and epistemic layers is essential for designing interventions that restore coherence, rebuild trust, and align public health strategies with lived experiences (see Appendix; Table 4).

Table 4: Summary of epistemological and ontological contributions of Lazzari and colleagues

Key Source	Observed Disruption	Strategic Insight / Conceptual Contribution
Lazzari et al. (2020a)	First psychiatric presentations during Covid-19: acute ontological distress	Psychiatry as frontline infrastructure; need for early intervention and ontological repair
Lazzari et al. (2020b)	Attempted mercy killing; existential collapse and relational fragmentation	Pandemic-induced psychosis as ontological rupture; clinical settings as sites of moral and epistemic crisis
Lazzari and Costigliola (1993a; 1993b)	Symbolic contagion and irrational intimacy in HIV transmission	Recognition of existential irrationalism; integration of moral reasoning into public health education
Lazzari, Gandolfi Colleoni, and Trallo (1996)	Psychosocial trauma and stigma in sexually transmitted diseases	Narrative repair and stigma-sensitive care; relational scaffolding for identity reconstruction
Lazzari and Masino (2015)	Public health foundations of health behaviour and meaning-making	Interdisciplinary health models: integration of phenomenology and ethics into clinical reasoning
Lazzari and Rabottini (2025a; 2025b)	Pandemic behaviours shaped by existential vulnerability and symbolic identity	Public health framework for health behaviour: integration of ethics, psychology, and public health strategy
Lazzari, Costley, and Nikolou-Walker (2024)	Epistemic closure and interpretive dominance in dyadic and group health narratives	Recognition of relational epistemology: implications for communication, teamwork, and symbolic resistance

CHAPTER 4

Epistemology of Pandemics

Introduction

Lazzari, Shoka, Nusair, and Rabottini (2020d) in 'Psychiatry in Time of Covid-19 Pandemic' (*Psychiatria Danubina*, 32(2): 229–235) highlight the psychiatric implications of the Covid-19 pandemic, emphasising how fear, isolation, and uncertainty destabilise mental health systems and individual psychological resilience. In Lazzari and colleagues (2020a), we examined the early psychiatric consequences of the Covid-19 crisis, focusing on clinical and systemic disruptions. The study identifies a pandemic as a multifaceted stressor that affects mental health through biological, psychological, and social pathways. It demonstrates that fear of infection, prolonged isolation, and media saturation contribute to increased anxiety, depression, and trauma-related symptoms across populations. A key finding is the emergence of acute psychiatric presentations, including pandemic-induced psychosis, as exemplified by a case of attempted suicide driven by delusional beliefs about Covid-19. This case illustrates how existential fear and symbolic contagion can fracture identity, distort moral reasoning, and lead to psychiatric emergencies.

We also critique the fragmentation of psychiatric services during the pandemic, noting that lockdowns and infection control measures might create some extra requirements for continuity of care, particularly for vulnerable groups, including older adults, people with pre-existing mental health conditions, and frontline healthcare workers. These facts call for adaptable, ethically grounded psychiatric responses that include telepsychiatry, community outreach, and trauma-informed care. Importantly, our research presents pandemics as ontological crises rather than merely biomedical ones. We argue that Covid-19 and any other pandemic crises can unsettle core assumptions about safety, agency, and relational meaning, requiring mental health services to engage with the existential aspects of suffering. We support a phenomenologically informed approach to mental health that recognises the symbolic, emotional, and moral dislocation experienced during global pandemic crises. In summary, Lazzari, Shoka, Nusair, and Rabottini (2020d) offer an early, interdisciplinary account of how pandemics reconfigure psychiatric practice, expose systemic vulnerabilities, and call for a re-evaluation of care models that address both clinical symptoms and deeper existential disruptions.

Epistemological foundations of pandemics

We critically examine the epistemological underpinnings of pandemic prevention by integrating public health knowledge with the interpretive complexities that arise during crises. We claim that, while disease-control methods—based on behavioural modelling, statistical inference, and predictive analytics—are essential for operational planning, they rely on implicit assumptions about human behaviour, social norms, and acceptable risk levels (Public Health England, 2020; Jatobá, Castro-Nunes, and de Carvalho, 2025). These assumptions become fragile under the psychological and social pressures of a pandemic. Drawing on findings from Lazzari and colleagues (2020a; 2020b; 2020c; 2020d), we postulate that pandemic lockdowns, uncertainty, and prolonged isolation undermine systems of trust, meaning-making, and perceptions of reality. For individuals with heightened vulnerability or diminished resilience, these disruptions precipitate emotional instability, behavioural dysregulation, and breakdowns in social relationships. The emergence of psychosis, suicidality, and conspiratorial thinking among populations facing pandemic threats signifies not only clinical deterioration but also a profound epistemological rupture in which the reliability of knowledge, authority, and self-understanding is questioned. In response, we advocate for public mental health strategies that are epistemically sensitive: approaches that incorporate care into emergency planning, restore interpretive coherence, and engage with layered belief systems that shape compliance and resistance. Such strategies should go beyond mere information provision to address the symbolic, emotional, and relational dimensions of pandemic response.

Public mental health during pandemic preparedness

Pandemics have often exposed a significant weakness in global and national public health strategies, especially in those geographical areas where implementation policies are slower: the marginalisation of psychiatry in preparedness planning. As Lazzari and colleagues (2020a; 2020b; 2020c; 2020d) demonstrated, individuals with pre-existing mental health conditions are not only more susceptible to psychological distress and clinical deterioration but also find it harder to adhere to public health measures, including isolation, hygiene protocols, and vaccination. These findings highlight the urgent need to prioritise public mental health as a fundamental component of pandemic preparedness, not merely a supplementary aspect of biomedical strategies but an essential part of the infrastructure. Incorporating psychosocial expertise into emergency planning, risk communication, and community resilience strategies is crucial to ensuring future responses are both clinically effective and ethically inclusive.

Policy action

Lazzari and colleagues (2020a; 2020b; 2020c; 2020d) offer critical insights that can directly inform policy development for future pandemic emergencies. Based on their findings, several actionable recommendations follow below.

Integrate psychiatric surge capacity into national emergency plans: Mental health services must be prepared to manage increases in psychiatric cases, including pandemic-induced psychoses, suicidality, anxiety, depression, paranoia (frequently, international conspiracy theories), and trauma-related conditions. This requires pre-arranged protocols, staffing reserves, and coordination with broader emergency infrastructure.

Implement simple, visual, and accessible communication methods for neurodivergent groups: Isolation and uncertainty disproportionately affect those with cognitive and communication differences. Public health messaging should be tailored using visual aids, plain language, and multimodal formats to promote inclusivity and understanding.

Allocate dedicated funding for mental health within pandemic preparedness budgets: Mental health must be recognised as essential infrastructure, not a secondary concern. Budget provisions should support telepsychiatry, community outreach, trauma-informed care, and the continuity of services for vulnerable groups.

These policy directions reflect the epistemic and clinical urgency emphasised by Lazzari, Shoka, Nusair, and Rabottini (2020d), positioning psychiatry as a vital pillar of ethically grounded, resilient pandemic-response systems.

Psychological distress as a public health indicator

Psychological distress must be recognised as an essential public health indicator, particularly during pandemics. Pandemic lockdowns, economic instability, and ongoing uncertainty significantly heighten anxiety, depression, and suicidality across populations. As Lazzari and colleagues (2020a; 2020b; 2020c; 2020d) demonstrated, these effects are unevenly distributed, with vulnerable and marginalised groups bearing the most significant burden because of pre-existing mental health issues, limited access to care, and intensified social stressors. In this context, psychosocial services serve as a societal early warning system—capable of detecting emerging patterns of psychological distress and guiding appropriate interventions. Incorporating psychiatric surveillance into public health infrastructure enables early identification of distress trends, promotes fair resource allocation, and supports the development of inclusive, trauma-informed strategies that address both clinical and systemic vulnerabilities.

Policy action

Building on Lazzari, Shoka, Nusair, and Rabottini (2020d) on pandemic mental health preparedness, the study provides a foundational framework for integrating psychiatric insights into pandemic policy. The findings support the following strategic actions:

- *Monitor mental health trends in real time:* Track helpline call volumes, psychotropic prescription rates, and engagement with digital mental health platforms to identify emerging distress patterns and support early intervention.
- *Deploy psychosocial support strategically:* Use data-driven indicators to target mental health resources to regions and populations experiencing heightened psychological strain, ensuring a targeted and equitable response.
- *Incorporate mental health metrics into surveillance systems:* Integrate psychiatric indicators into national and local epidemiological dashboards to align mental health monitoring with infectious disease surveillance, supporting comprehensive public health governance.

These measures recognise mental health as a vital part of pandemic infrastructure, thereby strengthening resilience, responsiveness, and ethical care across diverse communities.

Mental health equity and resilience as biosecurity

Reliable access to psychiatric care is not only a clinical necessity but also crucial for public health. During the Covid-19 pandemic, Lazzari and colleagues (2020a; 2020b; 2020c; 2020d) documented cases in which delayed psychiatric intervention led to acute hospitalisations and preventable complications, highlighting how mental health vulnerabilities can escalate into broader systemic risks. Individuals without prompt support may face crises that threaten personal well-being and undermine the effectiveness of public health measures, including isolation, vaccination, and hygiene protocols. To safeguard public health, psychiatric services must be recognised as essential infrastructure and remain fully operational during emergencies. This requires surge-capacity planning, continuity of care, and integration into broader biosecurity frameworks to ensure that mental health equity and resilience are incorporated into national preparedness strategies (Table 5).

Table 5: Summary table

Concept	Explanation	Application
Epistemology of Pandemics:	Pandemic prevention relies on behavioural models and statistical inference, but these are underpinned by fragile assumptions about human behaviour and social norms, particularly in crises.	Calls for epistemically attuned public health strategies that go beyond merely delivering data to address the emotional, symbolic, and relational aspects of knowledge and behaviour.
Public Mental Health:	Psychological interventions should not be marginalised during pandemic preparedness, as they play crucial roles in supporting vulnerable populations, shaping public health behaviours and knowledge, and ensuring compliance with health directives.	Reframe psychosocial interventions as a vital part of emergency infrastructure. Integrate psychiatric knowledge into risk communication and resilience plans for more inclusive and effective responses.
Policy Action:	Lazzari and colleagues (2020a; 2020b; 2020c; 2020d) suggest integrating mental health strategies into pandemic infrastructure by expanding surge capacity, promoting inclusive communication, and securing dedicated funding.	Develop protocols for psychiatric emergencies, adapt messaging for neurodivergent populations, and allocate resources for telepsychiatry and trauma-informed care.
Psychological Distress:	Psychological distress is a crucial public health indicator, particularly during pandemics. Vulnerable groups experience disproportionate impacts due to limited access and heightened stress.	Use psychiatric surveillance to identify distress trends, guide ethical resource allocation, and develop trauma-informed interventions. Integrate mental health metrics into epidemiological dashboards to support comprehensive governance.
Mental Health as Biosecurity:	Access to psychiatric care is essential for public health security. Delays in intervention can pose systemic risks and undermine adherence to health measures.	Recognise psychiatry as a vital component of biosecurity planning. Ensure ongoing care, surge capacity, and integration with wider emergency systems to safeguard individual well-being and public health.

Policy action

Building on the findings of Lazzari and colleagues (2020a; 2020b; 2020c; 2020d), the following policy actions are recommended to embed mental health equity in *pandemic preparedness.*

- *Legally recognise public (mental) health as essential infrastructure:* Emergency legislation should formally recognise psychiatric services as vital to national health policies and ongoing care, ensuring they remain operational during crises alongside other critical systems. For instance, it should designate a sentinel service to identify communities within the population that need additional support to adopt preventive behaviours.
- *Expand telepsychiatry, mobile clinics, and community-based models:* To sustain access during lockdowns or service disruptions, scalable and adaptable delivery models must be prioritised, particularly for underserved and remote populations. For example, expanding local services can help identify emotional and psychological barriers to adopting national preventive behaviours.
- *Include individuals with psychiatric conditions and neurodivergent individuals in emergency planning:* Simulation exercises and preparedness protocols should actively involve these groups to ensure that communication, logistics, and care strategies are inclusive, accessible, and ethically responsible. For example, include families of individuals who may face challenges with autonomy during pandemic restrictions.

These measures emphasise mental health as an essential component of biosecurity, resilience, and ethical public health governance, rather than treating it as a secondary issue.

Call to action

Lazzari and colleagues (2020a; 2020b; 2020c; 2020d) emphasise a clear imperative: mental health must be integrated into every stage of pandemic policy, from preparedness and response to recovery and resilience. Mental health and social services cannot remain marginal; they are frontline disciplines essential to safeguarding individual well-being and societal stability. Strengthening psychiatric infrastructure—through surge capacity, inclusive communication, and equitable access—improves public health outcomes and fosters social cohesion. Embedding psychosocial resilience into health governance is no longer optional; it is a strategic necessity for national and global security in future pandemics.

Epistemology of pandemic prevention and dissemination

We have examined the epistemological foundations of pandemic prevention by integrating public health knowledge with the interpretive complexities that emerge during crises. Epistemology—here understood as the phenomenological study of how knowledge is produced, justified, and legitimised—becomes particularly important in pandemics, where uncertainty, disruption, and contested authority converge. In the social sciences, epistemology shows how cultural norms, linguistic frameworks, and institutional logics shape what is regarded as valid knowledge (Carter and Little, 2007; Lehrer, 1990). These influences become even more evident during pandemics, where behavioural models, statistical forecasts, and predictive analytics, though vital, are underpinned by implicit assumptions about human behaviour, social values, and acceptable risks (Public Health England, 2020; Jatobá, Castro-Nunes, and de Carvalho, 2025). In the face of a global health crisis, these assumptions become epistemically fragile.

Building on Lazzari and colleagues (2020a; 2020b; 2020c; 2020d), we postulate that lockdowns, prolonged uncertainty, and social isolation weaken traditional trust systems, disrupt meaning-making, and unsettle perceptions of reality. For individuals with pre-existing mental health issues, emotional vulnerability, or limited social support, these disruptions lead to cognitive and interpersonal breakdowns, manifesting as epistemic confusion and resistance to public health measures. The rise in psychosis, suicidality, and conspiratorial beliefs during pandemic outbreaks reflects not only clinical decline but also a broader epistemological crisis in which the reliability of knowledge, the legitimacy of authority, and the coherence of self-understanding are all challenged.

These findings emphasise the urgent need for epistemically sensitive public mental health strategies. Such strategies should do more than disseminate information; they must address the interpretive and relational dimensions of crises. This entails engaging mental health professionals and social scientists in emergency planning, restoring interpretive stability, and engaging with the complex belief systems that shape public responses. Furthermore, these approaches need to consider the diverse health outcomes documented by scholars citing Lazzari and colleagues' work (Ahmad, 2020; Alsharji, 2022; Babicki et al., 2021; Becerra et al., 2021; Canpolat and Yildirim, 2021; Duman, 2021; Fancourt et al., 2021; Khan, 2021; Liu et al., 2021; Rania and Coppola, 2021). Doing so enables public health to develop a more resilient, inclusive, and epistemologically robust model of pandemic preparedness. Our contribution, 'Psychiatry in Time of COVID-19 Pandemic' (Lazzari et al., 2020d), has become a key element in reshaping the understanding of mental health within crisis governance. Scholars citing this work consistently regard it as a reference for illustrating the psychological impact of pandemic conditions, particularly the effects of uncertainty, isolation, and ethical strain on healthcare workers, students, and marginalised groups. These citations transcend clinical relevance, reinforcing the idea that psychosocial interventions must be proactively integrated into early warning systems and resilience frameworks rather than treated as reactive or secondary measures.

Our research has prompted a conceptual shift: public mental health is increasingly recognised not only as a therapeutic discipline but also as a vital component of pandemic preparedness and epistemic stability. This shift highlights the need to integrate mental health across all stages of emergency planning, including surveillance, communication, ethical triage, and recovery. As shown in Table 4, the academic consensus aligns with our findings, reflecting growing agreement that psychiatric insights are essential for safeguarding both individual well-being and the interpretative consistency of public health systems during crises.

Our publication 'Psychiatry in Time of Covid-19 Pandemic' (Lazzari et al., 2020d) has been cited by other authors to illustrate the psychiatric aspects of pandemic response. It has helped shape understanding of the psychological impact of uncertainty, isolation, and ethical dilemmas, particularly among healthcare workers, students, and marginalised populations. These citations reflect growing recognition that mental health is not a secondary concern but a vital part of crisis management. Monteith and colleagues (2021) highlighted increased psychiatric vulnerability to cybercrime during the pandemic, linking digital exposure to mental health risks. Sayeed and colleagues (2020) cited our work to demonstrate the psychiatric burden among adults with chronic illnesses, while Dongol and colleagues (2022) used it to illustrate the effect of Covid-19 on student sleep quality and stress levels.

Our findings have also been crucial in highlighting the psychological impact on frontline workers. Yilmaz, Erdogan, and Bahadir (2021) cited our study to document burnout and insomnia among healthcare staff, while Usul, Şan, and Bekgöz (2020) mentioned it to demonstrate anxiety among emergency medical personnel. Yasin and AlTamimi (2020) drew on our work to investigate the psychological framing of fear in the general population, and Matić, Takšić, and Božičević (2021) applied it to study resilience during concurrent crises, including earthquakes and the pandemic.

Further expanding its influence, Mahesar and colleagues (2023) quoted our study to analyse the psychiatric implications of lockdown and suicide reporting in the Pakistani media. Erjavac and colleagues (2023) used it to show an increase in acute psychiatric emergencies among children and adolescents, while Claus and colleagues (2022) mentioned it to highlight the long-term psychiatric consequences of ICU (intensive care unit) admission among Covid-19 patients. Collectively, these citations demonstrate how our research aligns with other authors' findings of the importance of redefining mental health and social services as crucial elements of pandemic preparedness, encouraging a shift towards incorporating psychosocial resilience into early warning systems and health governance (Table 6).

Table 6: Summary of the epistemology of pandemics.

Concept	Explanation	Application
Epistemology of Pandemic Prevention:	Inquiry into how knowledge is generated, justified, and legitimised, particularly in crisis conditions.	Guides the integration of mental health and social science into emergency planning and public health governance.
Knowledge Production and Legitimacy:	Shaped by cultural norms, linguistic structures, and institutional logics that define what counts as valid knowledge.	Explains how public health messaging and interventions are understood and trusted by diverse populations.
Operational Frameworks:	Behavioural models, statistical inference, and predictive analytics based on assumptions about conduct and risk.	Used in designing disease-control strategies, although susceptible to epistemic fragility during crises.
Crisis Conditions:	Situations of uncertainty, disruption, and contested authority that undermine normative systems of meaning.	Require adaptive, inclusive, and psychologically informed public health responses.
Epistemic Fragility:	Breakdown in the reliability of knowledge and authority under stress.	Leads to resistance to health measures, misinformation, and psychological distress.
Psychiatric Vulnerability:	Increased risk of psychosis, suicidality, and conspiratorial beliefs, particularly among emotionally or socially vulnerable individuals.	Requires early psychosocial interventions and ongoing psychiatric care in emergencies.
Interpretive Stability:	Restoration of coherent meaning-making and trust in knowledge systems.	Attained through inclusive communication, mental health support, and culturally sensitive public health strategies.
Policy Response:	Strategic incorporation of mental health into early warning systems, emergency legislation, and resilience frameworks.	Positions psychosocial interventions as a fundamental pillar of pandemic preparedness and of epistemic stability.

Pandemic epistemology must address irrationalism—not merely as a cognitive mistake, but as a phenomenological stance that treats emotion, instinct, and metaphysical beliefs as valid ways of understanding. Historical examples from the AIDS and Covid-19 pandemics show that people can act against their own interests even when they have accurate information about pandemic prevention (Lazzari et al., 1992; Goedert et al., 1995). This underlines the need to include psychological, cultural, and emotional factors in models of knowledge application, moving beyond purely rational assumptions (Dupré and Leonelli, 2022). Lazzari and colleagues (2020a; 2020b; 2020c; 2020d) describe severe psychotic episodes in individuals with no prior psychiatric history, triggered by fear, paranoia, and a sense of ontological collapse. Lazzari's concept of Samos Syndrome further expands this perspective, describing a form of pathophilia in which individuals intentionally expose themselves to transmissible diseases, including HIV, as symbolic or parasuicidal acts (Lazzari et al., 1991; Lazzari, 2023a).

As Lazzari and Costigliola (cited in La Rosa Nera, 2022) observe, these behaviours are challenging to influence through rational deterrence. They may be more common among individuals facing unresolved psychological challenges. In such circumstances, a pandemic and its associated risks can serve not only as external stressors but also as avenues for deeper emotional or existential struggles.

The danger itself becomes symbolically charged, providing a way to express deeper emotional and ontological tensions. According to Lazzari and colleagues (cited in Psicologi Italia, 2025), these behaviours are not impulsive but arise from deliberate, phenomenologically grounded choices. For some, such actions are perceived as socially meaningful or even heroic, embodying profound emotional resonance and a transcendent form of relational devotion. For some, intimacy can feel more profound—not despite the risk of infection, but partly because of it, with the closeness established carrying an emotional depth that surpasses normal boundaries (Lazzari, 1992). These insights challenge public health models based on rational compliance and highlight the importance of psychosocial approaches that consider the affective, cultural, and phenomenological aspects of behaviour. Alongside earlier analyses of symbolic illness narratives and psychosocial risk (Lazzari, Colleoni, and Trallo, 1995; Lazzari, Gandolfi Colleoni, and Trallo, 1996), we argue that irrationalism is central, not peripheral, to understanding human responses during pandemics. It demonstrates how pandemic crises evoke deep ontological and axiological tensions, in which non-rational forces influence decisions with significant social and ethical consequences.

Conclusions

Pandemics reveal the epistemological limits of public health systems, showing how pandemic crises disrupt not only biological and institutional frameworks but also the interpretive models through which people understand risk, authority, and relational meaning. From HIV/AIDS to Covid-19, irrationalism, symbolic behaviour, and epistemic confusion have become common responses to uncertainty rather than minor anomalies. These phenomena emphasise the need for prevention strategies that go beyond behavioural prediction and statistical modelling, favouring the integration of psychiatric care, cultural understanding, and ethical reasoning.

Samos Syndrome, as outlined by Lazzari and Rabottini (2022b; 2024a), provides a compelling framework for understanding such disruptions. It captures the irrational, emotionally charged behaviours that emerge during pandemics, particularly among individuals with emotional instability disorder. These behaviours, ranging from pathophilia (from ancient Greek: 'attraction to illness') to parasuicidal risk-taking, are not merely clinical curiosities but reflect more profound existential disorientation and symbolic engagement with contagion (Lazzari, 2023a; 2023b). By emphasising the lived experience of public health mandates and the embodied significance of pandemic rituals, pathophilia bridges psychiatric understanding and social theory, offering a model that is both diagnostically precise and conceptually sound.

The ethical implications of this framework are equally important. As Lazzari and Rabottini (2024a) argue, pandemic behaviours are ethically charged acts that reflect relational trauma, civic duty, and ontological vulnerability. High-risk actions and health behaviours may constitute acts of devotion, identity repair, or existential affirmation (Lazzari, 1992; 2023a; 2023b), challenging traditional narratives of compliance and responsibility. This view calls for a rethinking of public health ethics, moving away from individualised models of rational compliance towards relational paradigms of care, solidarity, and accountability.

The research by Lazzari and colleagues further supports this stance. Lazzari and colleagues (2020a; 2020b; 2020c; 2020d) documented psychosis and epistemic collapse during lockdown, advocating the integration of psychiatric care into emergency planning to restore interpretive stability. Lazzari and Costigliola (1993a; 1993b) examined deliberate HIV infection as a form of parasuicidal behaviour, highlighting the symbolic use of contagion and the need for phenomenological models in prevention. The evolving concept of Samos Syndrome (Lazzari et al., 1991; 2023) explores how metaphysical longing and pathophilic intimacy emerge under pandemic threat, emphasising the importance of cultural and affective insight for health policy.

Lazzari and Costigliola (cited in La Rosa Nera, 2022) analysed resistance to rational deterrence and interpreted contagion as an emotionally charged symbol, advocating the use of psychosocial frameworks to decode symbolic behaviour and existential struggles. In Psicologi Italia (2025), Lazzari and colleagues observed that public health decisions are perceived as heroic or redemptive acts, underscoring the need to integrate ethical reasoning into public health models. In the books *Water Lilies Adrift* and *Eros* (Lazzari, Colleoni, and Trallo, 1995; Lazzari et al., 1996), the authors addressed stigma and cultural narratives surrounding sexually transmitted diseases, supporting the incorporation of narrative medicine and stigma-sensitive communication. Finally, Lazzari (1992) examined how intimacy deepens under conditions of risk and recommended interventions tailored to relational and gendered contexts.

These insights support a multidimensional approach to pandemic preparedness—one that encompasses mental health equity, public health awareness, and psychosocial depth across all levels of governance. Mental health should be recognised as vital infrastructure, essential for restoring interpretive clarity, reducing distress, and fostering social resilience. Pathophilia and its related frameworks not only deepen our understanding of pandemic psychology but also expand the moral and epistemic vocabulary for interpreting, addressing, and ethically governing such behaviours.

CHAPTER 5

Axiology of Pandemics

Introduction

The study by Lazzari and colleagues (2020c) titled 'Clinical Psychopathology During Covid-19 Pandemic: Case Reports of First Psychiatric Presentations' examines how the Covid-19 pandemic triggered acute psychiatric episodes in individuals with no prior mental health history. Through case reports, the authors suggest that pandemic-related psychological stressors—such as isolation, fear of infection, and disruption of daily routines—can lead to severe psychopathological reactions, including psychosis, paranoia, and suicidal thoughts. The study emphasises that public health emergencies affect not only physical health but also mental health. The cases described reveal that existential uncertainty and social disconnection can disrupt the perception of reality and the maintenance of identity, resulting in first-time psychiatric episodes. These findings highlight the need to integrate mental health services into pandemic preparedness and response plans, treating psychiatric care as an essential part of infrastructure rather than a secondary concern.

This study offers a comprehensive psychological overview of how pandemics, particularly Covid-19, affect individuals and societies across interconnected domains. It begins by examining psychological vulnerability and adaptation, showing how invisible viral threats and prolonged social disruptions trigger widespread anxiety and uncertainty, with cognitive biases such as catastrophising and intolerance of uncertainty shaping public responses and health behaviours. The study then explores behavioural responses and compliance, highlighting how trust in institutions, perceived risk, and social norms influence adherence to public health measures such as mask-wearing and social distancing. Next, it discusses social cohesion and stigma, showing how pandemics can either strengthen or weaken social bonds, sometimes promoting solidarity, other times inciting scapegoating, xenophobia, and stigma against infected or marginalised groups. The research further investigates the mental health consequences of pandemics, emphasising long-term psychological impacts, including increased rates of depression, anxiety, PTSD (post-traumatic stress disorder), and burnout, particularly among healthcare workers and vulnerable populations. Finally, it considers the role of communication and misinformation, illustrating how inconsistent messaging and the spread of false information can erode public trust and foster harmful behaviours. Overall, these themes underline the importance of public health strategies that are not only scientifically sound but also psychologically considerate, ethically responsible, and culturally sensitive.

Pandemics' impact on the population and policies

Lazzari and colleagues' (2020a; 2020b; 2020c; 2020d) research advocates for supporting psychology research on pandemics by emphasising mental health as a crucial factor shaping public health behaviours and outcomes rather than an afterthought. It highlights that psychological preparedness—by fostering resilience, trust, and adaptive coping strategies—must be systematically incorporated into pandemic planning. From a policy perspective, we recommend integrating behavioural science into public health strategies, creating transparent, empathetic, and culturally sensitive communication campaigns, investing in mental health infrastructure as part of emergency preparedness, and monitoring psychosocial indicators alongside epidemiological data. We advocate a shift from reactive to proactive mental health policies during pandemic crises, recognising that how individuals think, feel, and act in such situations has significant implications for sociopsychological and political outcomes.

Since its publication, Lazzari and colleagues (2020a; 2020b; 2020c;

2020d) have been cited in studies examining the mental health impacts of Covid-19, particularly acute and first-onset psychiatric conditions. For instance, Rittmannsberger and colleagues (2022) cited it to support the hypothesis that psychosocial stressors, rather than direct viral infection, may trigger first-episode psychosis. Lazzari and colleagues (2020b) built directly on the original case series to emphasise the importance of early psychiatric recognition during pandemics.

Koca (2022) cited our study to highlight increased psychological vulnerability among young adults, thereby supporting the focus on emotional intelligence as a coping mechanism. Teo, Choo, and Tang (2024) used our findings as a benchmark for vaccine-related psychosis, situating their results within broader psychiatric patterns observed during the pandemic. Batteux, Taylor, and Carter (2021) incorporated our study into a systematic review to illustrate the clinical severity of pandemic-induced psychiatric conditions and to call for enhanced psychological support in future public health policies. Sehlikoğlu and Han Almiş (2022) cited our case series to support their hypothesis that pandemic-related stress increases the incidence of first-episode psychosis. Todorov, Avramova-Todorova, and Bureva (2023) cited our study to advocate for the inclusion of emotional intelligence training in higher education as a preventive measure against psychological decline. Overall, these citations demonstrate that the study has contributed to the ongoing discourse on the psychological effects of Covid-19, providing early descriptive data that has shaped both clinical and theoretical research across disciplines.

Axiology, affective ethics, and sacrificial logics in pandemic prevention

Axiology, the phenomenological study of values, offers a valuable lens for analysing moral reasoning during public health crises. As Pretorius (2024) notes, axiology encompasses both ethics—including justice, obligation, and virtue—and aesthetics, which relate to meaning, emotional connection, and the experience of beauty. In pandemics, ethical choices are often shaped not only by biomedical factors but also by personal, relational, and emotional considerations. Pandemic prevention involves morally significant decisions in which individuals frequently need to balance personal autonomy with collective welfare. Measures such as isolation, vaccination, and mask-wearing require relinquishing individual instincts for the sake of community safety. Lazzari and Rabottini (2025a; 2025b) introduced the concept of risk externalisation, demonstrating how private decisions—such as withholding symptom disclosure or vaccination status—can lead to public harm, transforming personal choices into collective consequences. Within close relationships, this dynamic becomes even more complex, as emotional bonds influence behaviour and moral judgement.

The importance of transparency and fairness in public health policy has been emphasised by Douglas (2009), while McClimans (2024) introduced the concept of dialogical ethics. This participatory approach treats prevention as a morally co-created practice that responds to diverse values and lived experiences. These approaches challenge top-down directives and promote ethical reasoning rooted in community dialogue and emotional insight. The implications of affective ethics have also been highlighted, particularly in the work of Lazzari and Masino (2015), who argued that perceptions of risk and behavioural responses are embedded in emotional and relational frameworks that cannot be addressed solely through rational appeals. Historical and psychosocial narratives further support this view. In their book *Water Lilies Adrift*, Lazzari, Colleoni, and Trallo (1995) examined how emotions such as love, danger, guilt, and liberation intertwine with ethical reasoning, demonstrating that vulnerability and desire are central to individuals' navigation of health disclosures and moral responsibility. The act of revealing one's health status—whether HIV-positive or experiencing symptoms during Covid-19—is hindered by fear of stigma and emotional consequences, despite its ethical importance.

Lazzari, Gandolfi Colleoni, and Trallo (1996) advanced bioethical discourse by advocating the inclusion of sacrificial logics, redefining harm, and recognising emotional and moral diversity. In the context of HIV/AIDS, Lazzari and Costigliola (1993a; 1993b) documented cases in which individuals engaged in unprotected sexual relationships across serological boundaries, often driven by fear of rejection and stigma. In these cases, infection was not perceived as harm but as a sacrificial act of love—an axiological inversion that reframed vulnerability as virtue and self-exposure as moral beauty. More specifically, HIV-negative persons having unprotected and consensual sexual relationships with HIV-positive individuals, and vice versa, HIV-positive persons hiding their HIV serological status from their sexual partners. Building on this, Lazzari and Rabottini (2024a) introduced Samos Syndrome to describe individuals—often those with personality disorders—who are drawn to relationships where they can become infected with HIV either through unprotected sexual relationships or close contacts with infected and contagious individuals. This behaviour has been understood as an ethical and emotional choice in which illness becomes a means of seeking closeness, meaning, or connection. The figure of the woman from Samos—an island once home to one of Europe's earliest leprosy infirmaries (Zambaco Pacha, 1981)—has been interpreted symbolically as representing compassion and solidarity rather than exclusion (Lazzari, Gandolfi Colleoni, and Trallo, 1996).

The pattern of citations demonstrates how the findings of Lazzari and colleagues (2020a; 2020b; 2020c) help to understand the affective and axiological disruptions produced by the pandemic. By documenting early psychiatric symptoms linked to uncertainty, isolation, and perceived threat, the study provided empirical accounts of how crises destabilise emotional regulation, value systems, and meaning-making processes. Subsequent research has extended these insights in multiple directions. Rittmannsberger and colleagues (2022) used our findings to support models in which psychosocial stressors precipitate psychosis, emphasising how heightened fear, social withdrawal, and existential threat can destabilise vulnerable individuals. Teo, Choo, and Tang (2024) applied the study to contextualise psychiatric reactions following Covid-19 vaccination, framing these responses within broader stress-related mechanisms rather than isolated adverse events. In educational psychology, Koca (2022) and Todorov, Avramova-Todorova, and Bureva (2023) cited the work to illustrate students' emotional strain, including anxiety, motivational decline, and cognitive overload. Their use of the study shows that the pandemic's axiological disruptions—loss of routine, uncertainty about the future, and diminished social meaning—affected learning environments as profoundly as clinical settings. Systematic reviews by Batteux, Taylor, and Carter (2021) further positioned our study into the broader evidence base on pandemic mental health, highlighting its contribution to mapping the severity and heterogeneity of psychiatric outcomes during Covid-19.

Together, these citations show that the affective and axiological frameworks underpinning the original study have informed clinical psychiatry, public health, educational psychology, and evidence synthesis. They collectively demonstrate how disruptions to values, emotional stability, and meaning shape individual behaviour and influence policy during pandemics (Table 7).

Table 7: Summative table

Theme	Conceptual Contribution	Implications for Pandemic Ethics
Axiology and Moral Reasoning:	Axiology, as defined by Pretorius (2024), encompasses ethics and aesthetics, providing a framework for understanding justice, obligation, emotional resonance, and meaning-making.	Ethical decisions during pandemics involve emotional and relational values beyond biomedical logic.
Risk Externalisation:	Lazzari and Rabottini (2025a; 2025b) introduced the concept to illustrate how private health decisions can result in collective harm.	Highlights the ethical complexity of balancing personal autonomy and public responsibility.
Dialogical and Community Ethics:	Douglas (2009) and McClimans (2024) advocate participatory ethics that are responsive to diverse values and lived experiences.	Supports inclusive, transparent public health policies grounded in community dialogue.
Affective Ethics:	Lazzari and Masino (2015) emphasise that emotional and relational contexts shape risk perception and behaviour.	Ethical frameworks must incorporate the emotional and symbolic dimensions of decision-making.
Sacrificial Logics and Moral Inversion:	Lazzari and Costigliola (1993a; 1993b) and Lazzari, Gandolfi Colleoni, and Trallo (1996) document cases in which infection is regarded as a sacrificial act of love.	Reframes vulnerability as a virtue and self-exposure as moral beauty.

Theme	Conceptual Contribution	Implications for Pandemic Ethics
Samos Syndrome:	Lazzari and Rabottini (2024a) describe a syndrome in which individuals seek relationships with infected or marginalised partners.	Illness becomes a route to emotional intimacy and to existential meaning.
Historical Symbolism:	Zambaco Pacha (1981) and Lazzari et al. (1996) describe the Samos leprosy infirmary as a model of solidarity.	Provides historical precedent for the ethics of inclusion and relational care.
Psychiatric Case Studies:	Lazzari et al. (2020a; 2020b; 2020c; 2020d) documented first-onset psychiatric cases during Covid-19, as cited by Rittmannsberger et al. (2022), Teo, Choo, and Tang (2024), Koca (2022), Todorov, Avramova-Todorova, and Bureva (2023), and Batteux, Taylor, and Carter (2021).	Validates the role of affect and psychosocial stress in shaping mental health and ethical behaviour during pandemics.

Conclusions

The axiological implications of our research indicate that ethical reasoning during pandemics cannot rely solely on biomedical logic. Evidence shows that values such as vulnerability, relational fidelity, emotional closeness, and sacrificial care are essential to how individuals make moral decisions in crises. By emphasising affective and existential aspects, our studies challenge dominant paradigms that prioritise invulnerability, autonomy, and rationality. Instead, we support a pluralistic moral landscape—one in which suffering is not merely something to be avoided but a space for ethical engagement, solidarity, and meaning-making. This reframing encourages the development of more inclusive and emotionally sensitive bioethics, capable of addressing the complexities of human experience during periods of deep uncertainty that emerge during pandemic outbreaks and in their repercussions (Table 8).

Table 8: Axiological implications of pandemic ethics in Lazzari and colleagues' research

Key Source	Observed Axiological Disruption	Strategic Integration
Lazzari et al. (2020a; 2020b; 2020c; 2020d)	Collapse of moral coherence and psychiatric stability during lockdown; epistemic confusion.	Embed psychiatric care within emergency planning; restore interpretive and moral stability.
Lazzari and Rabottini (2025a; 2025b)	Private moral decisions producing collective harm; ethical tension in intimate relationships.	Reframe prevention as relational ethics; integrate moral reasoning into public health mandates.
Douglas (2009); McClimans (2024)	Erosion of trust due to top-down mandates and the exclusion of plural moral voices.	Promote dialogical ethics; embed transparency and fairness in participatory health policymaking.
Lazzari and Masino (2015); Ceronetti (1993)	Emotional ambivalence and affective dissonance in risk perception; neglect of existential suffering.	Recognise affective ethics; integrate poetic and humanistic models into health communication.
Lazzari, Colleoni, and Trallo (1995)	Disclosure dilemmas are shaped by fear, stigma, and emotional fallout.	Address vulnerability as an ethical strength; support relational disclosure through stigma-sensitive frameworks.
Lazzari, Gandolfi Colleoni, and Trallo (1996)	Sacrificial ethics and moral inversion; redefinition of harm and virtue.	Expand bioethical discourse to include sacrificial logics; honour emotional and moral plurality.
Lazzari and Costigliola (1993a; 1993b)	Infection as an allegedly intentional moral act; resistance to biomedical deterrence.	Interpret irrationalism as an ethical expression; embed public health reasoning into prevention models.
Lazzari and Rabottini (2024a; 2024b)	Illness as a conduit for intimacy; relational fidelity privileged over self-preservation.	Reconfigure vulnerability as a moral choice; integrate sacrificial ethics into relational care models.
Zambaco Pacha (1981); Lazzari et al. (1996)	Historical solidarity over exclusion: marriage between infected persons and healthy individuals.	Use historical-poetic emblems to inspire inclusive ethics; elevate relational fidelity within health policy.
Lazzari et al. (2020a; 2020b; 2020c; 2020d); Koca (2022); Todorov, Avramova-Todorova, and Bureva (2023); Batteux, Taylor, and Carter (2021)	Emotional strain and psychiatric vulnerability across populations; fragmentation of moral resilience.	Strengthen psychological support within preparedness frameworks; align mental health with axiological insight.

CHAPTER 6

Impact of Pandemics on Society and Education

Introduction

The study by Lazzari, McAleer, Nusair, and Rabottini (2021) titled 'Psychiatric Training During the COVID-19 Pandemic Benefits from Integrated Practice in Interprofessional Teams and Ecological Momentary e-Assessment' examines how psychiatric education adapted to the challenges of the Covid-19 pandemic through innovative, collaborative, and technology-driven methods. The authors argue that the disruption of traditional face-to-face training prompted a shift towards integrated learning models that combined interprofessional teamwork with real-time digital assessment. Specifically, the study introduces Ecological Momentary e-Assessment (EMeA), a mobile-based tool that enables students to record their clinical experiences, emotional responses, and learning reflections in real time. This approach not only helps minimise recall bias but also provides continuous feedback and emotional monitoring, which are especially valuable during periods of heightened stress and uncertainty.

The research involved 228 students from various healthcare disciplines, including psychiatry, medicine, nursing, psychology, and physiotherapy, organised into interprofessional teams. The findings show that these collaborative environments improved clinical outcomes, increased patient satisfaction, and fostered mutual respect among trainees. Psychiatric trainees, in particular, benefited from exposure to complex cases requiring coordinated care, especially those involving Covid-19 patients with comorbid mental health conditions. The study highlights how interprofessional education (IPE) enhances teamwork, communication, and ethical sensitivity—skills vital in crises, where quick decision-making and emotional resilience are essential.

Furthermore, the use of EMeA enabled educators to observe students' emotional states, including stress, mindfulness, and satisfaction, thereby integrating affective aspects into the learning process. This aligns with broader axiological and affective ethical frameworks that emphasise emotional closeness, relational fidelity, and reflective practice in moral decision-making. The authors report statistically significant improvements in students' attitudes towards interprofessional collaboration, with 73% agreeing that IPE skills could be transferred to daily practice and 77% of patients recognising the benefits of integrated care. In the context of pandemic preparedness and response, the study shows that university training can be sustained and even improved through digital innovation and team-based learning. It advocates including mobile assessment tools and interprofessional models in future educational programmes, ensuring that trainees are equipped not only with clinical skills but also with emotional awareness and ethical flexibility.

Pandemic disruption in education, society, and social integration

The Covid-19 pandemic caused significant disruptions to education, professional collaboration, and social integration, transforming how people learn, interact, and connect with institutions. In this context, Lazzari and colleagues (2021) provide a detailed account of how psychiatric training adapted to crisis conditions, highlighting broader implications for educational resilience and interprofessional practice. The study shows that lockdowns and travel restrictions limited access to clinical placements and face-to-face instruction, prompting institutions to adopt digital platforms such as Microsoft Teams and Zoom and to implement a hybrid educational model. This model includes Ecological Momentary e-Assessment—a real-time, context-aware tool that enabled students to record emotional, cognitive, and behavioural responses during training. The system, which remains active and evolving, allows educators to monitor learners' progress and emotional well-being, offering a flexible alternative to traditional evaluation methods.

This shift reflects a broader pedagogical shift towards hybrid learning environments that combine digital and face-to-face methods to maintain continuity during emergencies and beyond. Gervasi, Müller, and Reiter (2022) observed that the pandemic accelerated the development of secure electronic assessment systems, while Kaap-Fröhlich, Müller, and Reimann (2022) supported integrating interprofessional education (IPE) into national curricula through digitally adaptable frameworks. These developments align with wider public health strategies focused on decentralisation, digital inclusion, and responsiveness (Public Health England, 2020). The digitisation of medical education, as discussed in Lazzari and colleagues (2021), exemplifies these strategies by promoting collaborative, real-time learning across disciplines.

Pandemics also reshaped the meaning of social integration in educational and cultural contexts. Restrictions on physical gatherings curtailed participation in academic and community events, prompting a re-evaluation of how inclusion and engagement are promoted. In this context, Lazzari's research contributes to a growing body of evidence supporting the integration of digital tools, emotional monitoring, and interprofessional collaboration as vital components of resilient education systems capable of withstanding future public health crises.

Interprofessional collaboration and social reconfiguration

Pandemics prompt significant reorganisation of interprofessional collaboration and social learning, particularly in medical education. As interprofessional education (IPE) typically relies on face-to-face interaction, it may rapidly shift to digital formats, enabling students and educators to connect via mobile apps and remote platforms (Lazzari et al., 2021). These synchronous and asynchronous, device-independent interactions sustain mentorship and peer support despite the spatial separation caused by lockdowns and distancing measures. Rather than weakening collaborative learning, this shift fosters new forms of digital solidarity, enabling participants to maintain relational depth and professional accountability in virtual settings.

The use of tools such as Ecological Momentary e-Assessment (EMeA) is central to this transformation. Chew, Maniam, and Sim (2024) emphasise the importance of real-time, context-sensitive evaluation methods in health education and IPE, noting that instruments such as EMeA are essential for capturing behavioural and reflective learning outcomes. These tools enable continuous monitoring of emotional and cognitive responses, providing a more nuanced understanding of student development. Hatamnejad, Farhadi, and Zarei (2023) also examined the psychological impact of pandemic-era training, finding that emotional intelligence and structured digital reflection can help prevent burnout and enhance well-being. This insight aligns with Lazzari, Costley, and Nikolou-Walker (2024), who advocate reflective practice as a key element of professional growth and resilience.

These educational adaptations reflect broader societal shifts in how technology mediates connection, meaning, and relationships. As Butler (2022) argues, a pandemic may prompt a realignment of everyday life, with shared vulnerability and interdependence central to personal and professional relationships. The digitalisation of interprofessional collaboration not only sustains learning during a pandemic and students' distancing from university campuses but also transforms how solidarity, empathy, and ethical engagement are cultivated across disciplines through digital platforms.

Transformation of routine social interactions

The transformation of routine social interactions during pandemics extends beyond institutional settings and profoundly affects everyday life. Remote work, greater reliance on digital technologies, and mobility restrictions significantly alter how people interact, learn, and connect. The closure of public spaces and the widespread shift to home-based environments disrupt familiar daily routines and blur the lines between public and private spheres (Cambridge Dictionary, 2025a; Merriam-Webster Dictionary, 2025). These changes show how pandemics reshape not only education and employment systems but also the experience of social integration, prompting reflection on what it means to be present, connected, and professionally engaged during times of crisis.

Ritunnano and colleagues (2023) examined this reconfiguration through a phenomenological lens, demonstrating that health behaviours must be understood as emotional and relational adaptations. Their perspective aligns with findings from Lazzari and colleagues (2021), whose study of psychiatric training during the pandemic shows that students' emotional states and interpersonal dynamics are significantly affected by the absence of in-person tutors and reliance on digital platforms. The shift to virtual learning environments, although necessary, introduces new forms of isolation and emotional stress, highlighting the need for educational models that foster relational closeness and emotional well-being. Together, these insights reveal that pandemic-era adaptations have altered the meaning of social presence, emphasising the importance of vulnerability, interdependence, and emotional connection in both personal and professional spheres through alternative social platforms, including digital spaces.

Ontology, epistemology, and axiology of pandemics' impact on Society

It has been observed that pandemics significantly influence emotional states, which in turn affect public rationality. In an earlier work (Lazzari, 2020), it is argued that the ability to reason and its translation into preventative behaviours are heavily affected by fear, uncertainty, and social context. This emotional-cognitive interaction indicates that public responses to health crises are not merely scientific or procedural; instead, they are rooted in the relational and emotional aspects of human experience.

Axiology: Reframing societal values during pandemics

Pandemics are pivotal moments that prompt a profound reassessment of societal values and ethical priorities. They expose the limitations of purely rationalist models in shaping health-related behaviours, particularly during periods of emotional stress and systemic upheaval. In this context, our research (Lazzari and Rabottini, 2024a) underlines the importance of values such as solidarity, emotional resilience, and adaptability. These affective and relational qualities—often intuitive and impulsive—are crucial in shaping both individual and collective responses to crises. This axiological transformation challenges the supremacy of cognition, indicating that ethical behaviour under pressure is often influenced by emotional intelligence and relational factors.

This perspective is reflected in the GMA Committee's Position Paper (Kaap-Fröhlich, Müller, and Reimann, 2022), which cites our work to support the integration of interprofessional education (IPE) into national curricula. In this context, IPE is not merely a pedagogical innovation but an ethical response to systemic fragility. It fosters collaborative skills that emphasise emotional awareness and shared responsibility. During a pandemic, digital collaboration emerged not only as a logistical solution but as a moral necessity, embodying a renewed ethical consciousness centred on proximity, care, and adaptive solidarity.

Hatamnejad, Farhadi, and Zarei (2023) further developed this ethical perspective by citing our work to argue that reflective mobile learning can help reduce emotional fatigue and stress. In disrupted educational settings, relational health behaviour is regarded as a collective ethical duty rather than merely a personal benefit. This view aligns with core principles in public health ethics, particularly those influenced by Dewey's pragmatism (Dewey, 1925; 1927; 1939) and the normative frameworks of Thompson and Upshur (Thompson and Upshur, 2017; Upshur, 2002). These traditions emphasise justice, vulnerability, and relational accountability, values that pandemics starkly highlight. Our research supports these ideas by showing that educational reform must be behaviourally responsive and grounded in normative reasoning that addresses both the emotional and relational aspects of human experience. Similarly, higher education becomes a preferred platform for preparing academics and students for pandemic preparedness by integrating cognitive skills into predictive tasks.

Embedding pandemic preparedness in higher education

Pandemic preparedness is a global imperative, yet higher education institutions remain underutilised in embedding resilience, interdisciplinary knowledge, and adaptive skills into curricula. Universities are uniquely placed to cultivate public health literacy, ethical leadership, and systems innovation. We propose a framework for integrating pandemic preparedness into higher education, emphasising curricular design, research priorities, institutional resilience, and policy alignment. By embedding preparedness across teaching, research, and community engagement, higher education can act as a proactive agent in safeguarding well-being, advancing innovation, and reinforcing collective responsibility. The chapter outlines the theoretical foundations, practical strategies, and implications for policy and practice.

The Covid-19 pandemic revealed profound vulnerabilities across health systems, economies, and societies. While governments and healthcare providers bore the immediate burden of the response, universities contributed by rapidly shifting to online learning, conducting vaccine research, and disseminating public health information (Iglesias-Pradas et al., 2021). Yet these efforts were largely reactive, reflecting the absence of a systematic preparedness framework within higher education. Embedding pandemic preparedness into universities' missions is therefore essential. Higher education institutions are incubators of interdisciplinary knowledge and critical thinking, preparing graduates to navigate crises across sectors (Visvizi, Nawaz, and Kozłowski, 2023).

Preparedness in higher education can be understood through resilience theory, systems thinking, and ethical governance. Resilience theory emphasises the need for universities to build adaptive capacity, enabling students and staff to anticipate, absorb, and recover from disruptions (Nandy, Lodh, and Tang, 2021). Systems thinking highlights the interconnectedness of health, economic, educational, and social systems, underlining that pandemics are not isolated health events but crises that ripple across every domain of society (Celbis, van de Laar, and Volante, 2023). Ethical governance emphasises cultivating values of equity, transparency, and collective responsibility, ensuring that preparedness initiatives are socially just as well as technically sound (Crawford, 2023).

Embedding preparedness requires deliberate curricular innovation that transcends traditional disciplinary boundaries. Public health literacy must be integrated across programmes, ensuring that students in business, engineering, the social sciences, and the arts understand the fundamentals of epidemiology, infection control, and health communication (Jumaa et al., 2023). Interdisciplinary learning should be encouraged, enabling students to collaborate across faculties to address the multifaceted nature of pandemics. Simulation and scenario-based learning can provide students with opportunities to practise crisis decision-making. At the same time, ethics and leadership modules can prepare them to confront dilemmas of resource allocation, equity, and governance during times of crisis.

Research and innovation

Universities are engines of discovery, and embedding preparedness requires aligning research agendas with global health priorities. Biomedical research into vaccines and therapeutics remains essential. Still, it must be complemented by advances in digital health and data analytics that enable modelling of disease spread and the informed development of policy (Visvizi, Nawaz, and Kozłowski, 2023). Social and behavioural research is equally critical, as understanding public compliance, misinformation, and cultural factors can determine the success or failure of interventions (Celbis, van de Laar, and Volante, 2023). Policy translation must be prioritised to ensure that research findings are communicated effectively to policymakers and practitioners.

Preparedness must extend beyond curricula and research into the operational and didactic structures of universities and higher education. Institutions must establish crisis management protocols to guarantee continuity of teaching, research, and student support during disruptions (Nandy, Lodh, and Tang, 2021). Investment in digital infrastructure is essential to ensure robust platforms for online learning and collaboration (Iglesias-Pradas et al., 2021). Universities should engage actively with their communities, partnering with local health systems to disseminate information and provide support during crises (Jumaa et al., 2023). Global collaboration is equally important, as networks with international institutions enable the sharing of resources and knowledge (Visvizi, Nawaz, and Kozłowski, 2023).

Embedding preparedness in higher education has significant implications for policy and practice. Governments must recognise universities as key partners in preparedness planning and integrate them into national strategies (Crawford, 2023). Accreditation bodies can mandate the inclusion of preparedness competencies in curricula, ensuring consistency across institutions. Funding streams should support research and curricular innovation, while policies must address equity and access to ensure preparedness initiatives do not exacerbate existing disparities (Celbis, van de Laar, and Volante, 2023).

Several universities have begun embedding preparedness into their structures, offering valuable examples of feasibility and impact. Some institutions have introduced pandemic modules in public health and business programmes, while others have established interdisciplinary centres for infectious disease research (Visvizi, Nawaz, and Kozłowski, 2023). Collaborations with local health authorities have enabled universities to deliver vaccination campaigns and public education initiatives (Jumaa et al., 2023). These cases demonstrate that embedding preparedness is both achievable and beneficial, providing models that can be adapted and scaled across diverse contexts.

Challenges and limitations

Embedding preparedness is not without challenges. Resource constraints may limit universities' ability to implement new curricula or research initiatives (Nandy, Lodh, and Tang, 2021). Resistance to change can arise when faculty and administrators prioritise traditional disciplines over emerging needs. Global disparities mean that institutions in low-resource settings face greater barriers to preparedness (Celbis, van de Laar, and Volante, 2023). Sustainability is another concern, as ensuring that preparedness initiatives remain embedded beyond immediate crises requires long-term commitment (Crawford, 2023).

Future efforts must focus on developing global frameworks that establish international standards for preparedness curricula (Visvizi, Nawaz, and Kozłowski, 2023). Technology integration will be critical, with artificial intelligence, simulation, and digital platforms offering new opportunities for teaching and research (Iglesias-Pradas et al., 2021). Interprofessional education should be expanded to train students across disciplines to collaborate effectively in crisis response (Jumaa et al., 2023). Evaluation and metrics must be established to assess the effectiveness of preparedness initiatives, ensuring accountability and continuous improvement (Celbis, van de Laar, and Volante, 2023).

Pandemic preparedness must be embedded in higher education to build resilient societies and informed professionals. Universities are uniquely placed to integrate interdisciplinary knowledge, foster adaptive skills, and promote ethical governance. By embedding preparedness across curricula, research, and institutional structures, higher education can act as a proactive agent in safeguarding well-being, advancing innovation, and reinforcing collective responsibility. While challenges remain, the opportunities for higher education to contribute to global resilience are profound. Embedding pandemic preparedness is not merely academic; it is a moral imperative for the future of global health.

Ontology: Redefining the meaning of learning and social interaction

Pandemics undermine the ontological foundations of education and social life, requiring a redefinition of learning and relational engagement. Learning can no longer be viewed as a static, classroom-bound event; instead, it must be understood as a dynamic, embodied process—fluid, situated, and responsive to broader social contexts. This reconceptualisation was developed by Lazzari, McAleer, Nusair, and Rabottini (2021), who framed learning as an adaptive interaction with lived reality, shaped by emotional, spatial, interpersonal, global, and technological contingencies.

Chew, Maniam, and Sim (2024) cited Lazzari, McAleer, Nusair, and Rabottini (2021) in their use of Ecological Momentary e-Assessment (EMeA) via digital platforms, endorsing it as a method for capturing interprofessional practice in medical training. EMeA's capacity to record lived experiences in real time highlights the move towards experiential, context-aware learning. This shift reflects broader pandemic-related changes in educational practices: remote work, reliance on digital technology, and disrupted routines have transformed how people collaborate, communicate, and learn. Furthermore, the acquisition and endorsement of pandemic-related data are dynamic and continually seek to fill knowledge gaps.

Gervasi, Müller, and Reiter (2022) also cited Lazzari and colleagues' work to support decentralised, secure digital assessment infrastructures. This shift signals a move away from institutionalised evaluation towards mobile, flexible, and ethically responsive engagement. In this new landscape, learning is not only a cognitive activity but also an ontological and ethical response to pandemic uncertainty—demanding presence, adaptability, and emotionally attuned interactions across digital and embodied realms.

Guerrero Fernandez (2022) expands this ontological perspective by introducing the concept of ontological stratification, arguing that pandemics should be understood as layered phenomena encompassing biological, social, and existential dimensions. These layers interact through contingency and vulnerability, showing that pandemic ontology is not a single truth but a constellation of conditions that shape life across different domains. This framework is supported by research demonstrating that educational and emotional realities are co-produced within lived spaces—bodies, homes, and institutions—rather than confined to clinical or academic silos.

This layered understanding becomes increasingly urgent as solipsism—the philosophical view that only one's own mind is sure to exist—resurfaces during prolonged social isolation and disrupted intersubjective contact (Merriam-Webster, 2024; Encyclopaedia Britannica, 2024b). Such an existential reorientation prompts deeper ontological and epistemological reflection, challenging the foundations of collective responsibility. Solipsism undermines mutual recognition, which is essential for effective public health. It creates a gap between propositional knowledge ('knowing what'), practical knowledge ('knowing how'), and embodied conviction ('believing what'). As Lazzari and Rabottini (2025a; 2025b) show, this divide often manifests as resistance to public health interventions, highlighting the need for educational reform that is not only cognitively rigorous but also emotionally and relationally grounded.

The definition of irrational health behaviour during a pandemic—any action that increases personal risk despite awareness of the illness and its consequences (Lazzari and Costigliola, 1993a; 1993b)—aligns with medical capacity assessments (NHS, 2024). These assessments comprise four main components: understanding risk, retaining information, weighing decisions, and communicating choices. Disruption in any of these components can result in incomplete capacity and reduced prevention. The ontological turn offers a useful interpretive lens for understanding such behaviours: to understand health-related decision-making in pandemic contexts, one must explore the metaphysical tradition of irrationalism, which emphasises intuition, volition, and emotion over rational thinking (Encyclopaedia Britannica, 2024a).

Epistemology: Rethinking knowledge in pandemic conditions

Pandemic conditions demand a rethinking of epistemology—specifically, how knowledge is created, validated, and shared. Retrospective abstraction and institutional certainty, long regarded as foundational to educational and scientific authority, are increasingly questioned. In response, a digital education framework is introduced that prioritises immediacy, emotional insight, and contextual responsiveness, reflecting the pandemic's complex realities. This epistemic shift redefines knowledge as contingent, embodied, and relational rather than static or universally transferable. Chew, Tan, and Ong (2024) operationalised this framework to structure outcome-based evaluations in medical and nursing education, emphasising real-time, experience-sensitive metrics. Gervasi, Müller, and Reiter (2022) also drew on our research to design scalable digital infrastructures that support decentralised, emotionally attuned learning environments. Hatamnejad, Farhadi, and Zarei (2023) applied similar principles to emotional well-being research, while Kaap-Fröhlich, Müller, and Reimann (2022) integrated its concepts into policy-level curriculum reform. These applications exemplify a broader shift in educational epistemology—where knowledge emerges through adaptive engagement, ethical responsiveness, and the co-creation of meaning across disrupted, digitised, and emotionally charged contexts. The same occurs on a larger scale across societies and countries facing pandemic threats. Knowledge and understanding are socially constructed and deconstructed at a rapid pace, depending on ever-changing data related to pandemic spread. This process is then integrated into social learning and behaviour to produce the expected or unexpected societal response to a pandemic.

This body of work questions traditional views of knowledge sharing and creation during pandemic restrictions, highlighting a significant epistemological shift. Before a pandemic, knowledge is typically regarded as stable, shareable, and confirmed through social consensus, grounded in institutional authority or the sedimentation of multiple realities over time. However, pandemics disrupt these foundations, replacing certainty with ambiguity, urgency, and emotional pressure. In this altered landscape, knowledge production becomes more solitary and self-directed. Individuals are compelled to make critical decisions—about health, relationships, and ethics—relying on incomplete information, disputed truths, and rapidly changing data. A pandemic, especially during its initial moments and the outbreak of new infected cases, encourages multiple epistemologies, in which diverse and sometimes conflicting truths coexist. This shift challenges conventional ideas of rational debate and expert authority, emphasising the importance of contingency, emotion, and embodied experience in shaping what is recognised as knowledge. In such circumstances, knowledge is not simply transmitted; it is negotiated, improvised, and emotionally charged. It occurs within lived spaces and disrupted routines, often bypassing formal channels and institutional gatekeeping. This new perspective has significant implications for education, public health, and ethical decision-making, stressing the need for frameworks that accept uncertainty, decentralised reasoning, and the relational nature of knowing.

The epistemological complexity of pandemic contexts is further emphasised by Nie, Zhang, and Li (2021), who found that individuals may ignore public health guidance even when they understand the associated risks. This behavioural inconsistency challenges normative definitions of rationality—usually described as decision-making based on clear thought and reason (Cambridge Dictionary, 2025b)—and highlights the emotionally driven, socially embedded nature of human action under psychosocial stress. As argued by Lazzari and Rabottini (2025a; 2025b), effective public health responses require not only epidemiological accuracy but also a nuanced understanding of the psychosocial and behavioural dynamics that influence compliance, resilience, learning, and knowledge. A body of research highlights the importance of closely examining the pedagogical benefits of studying pandemics. In situations marked by urgency, risk, catastrophe, and disaster, a widening gap emerges between collective, shareable knowledge—such as interprofessional learning and collaborative practice—and solipsistic epistemologies, characterised by personal, autonomous worldviews that remain unexamined by peers. This divergence reflects the tension between socially validated knowledge and individually constructed meaning, a tension often heightened by isolation and emotional strain, as occurs during pandemic lockdowns.

To address this epistemic fragmentation, educational models should be designed to harmonise individual cognition with collective ethical engagement. Learning must remain socially responsive and epistemologically inclusive, integrating multiple perspectives and fostering shared responsibility. Such models should honour the relational nature of knowing, accommodate emotional and contextual differences, and support the co-creation of meaning in disrupted and digitised environments. This approach ensures that knowledge remains not only valid and actionable but also ethically grounded and socially attuned.

Contributions of our research findings

The impact of our research on interprofessional education, digital assessment, and emotionally attuned learning frameworks has been cited in several publications, each of which extends our conceptual and methodological contributions into new areas of practice and policy. Our findings informed policy discussions on incorporating interprofessional education (IPE) into national medical curricula, particularly amid the digital constraints imposed by the Covid-19 pandemic. In this context,

IPE was redefined not merely as a pedagogical reform but as a structural response to systemic fragility. This development requires collaborative skills and emotional intelligence in digitally mediated environments.

Chew, Maniam, and Sim (2024) incorporated our clinically validated model, the Ecological Momentary e-Assessment (EMeA), into their scoping review of interprofessional education interventions in mental healthcare. By operationalising EMeA, they demonstrated how clinical training can be assessed using real-time, context-aware metrics that reflect lived experiences and interprofessional dynamics. This application emphasised the importance of experience-sensitive tools in mental health education.

Gervasi, Perri, and Simonetti (2022) drew on our research in their study, 'Strategies and System Implementations for Secure Electronic Written Exams'. Our work provided a real-world example of mobile-based, secure digital assessment, supporting their argument for decentralised exam systems that are scalable, resilient, and ethically responsive to pandemic-induced disruptions. Hatamnejad, Farhadi, and Zarei (2023) cited our research in their multicentre study 'Emotional Intelligence and Happiness in Clinical Medical Students'. Our theoretical contributions supported the use of reflective mobile learning as a buffer against emotional fatigue and stress in disrupted educational environments. This citation affirmed the relevance of our work in promoting emotional resilience and well-being among medical trainees.

Finally, the study 'The Assessment of Interprofessional Practice in Mental Health Nursing with Ethnographic Observation and Social Network Analysis' (Lazzari, McAleer, Rabottini, 2022) directly extends our research. It advocates EMeA as an evaluative tool for interprofessional collaboration, combining ethnographic and mixed-methods approaches to capture the complexity of mental health nursing practice. This work demonstrates the ongoing development of our framework within UK NHS Trusts and academic centres. Collectively, these studies show how conceptual innovations—particularly those addressing immediacy, emotional insight, and decentralised learning—have influenced policy, pedagogy, and clinical training across diverse cultural and institutional settings.

Conclusions

Pandemics are transformative forces that reshape human values, social realities, and modes of knowing. Axiologically, they expose the limits of rigid institutional norms and foreground solidarity, emotional resilience, and adaptability as core ethical commitments. Interprofessional education becomes a moral obligation rather than a logistical choice, as articulated in the GMA Committee's Position Paper (Kaap-Fröhlich, Müller, and Reimann, 2022). Reflective mobile learning, as shown by Hatamnejad, Farhadi, and Zarei (2023), operates as an ethical mechanism for sustaining emotional well-being and promoting rational, health-oriented behaviour as a shared moral resource. Ontologically, pandemics destabilise inherited assumptions about learning and social interaction, positioning education as an embodied, adaptive, and relational process, as proposed in the EMeA model (Lazzari et al., 2021) and later affirmed in psychiatric training by Chew, Maniam, and Sim (2024). This shift is reinforced by decentralised digital infrastructures (Gervasi, Müller, and Reiter, 2022) and by Guerrero Fernandez's (2022) account of ontological stratification, which frames pandemics as layered phenomena spanning biological, social, and existential dimensions. These perspectives converge to show that educational and emotional life are co-constructed within lived spaces—homes, bodies, and institutions—while the resurgence of solipsistic tendencies during isolation (Merriam-Webster, 2024; Encyclopaedia Britannica, 2024b) demonstrates how weakened intersubjectivity erodes collective responsibility and intensifies the need for relational, embodied learning. Epistemologically, pandemics reconfigure how knowledge is generated and validated, privileging immediacy, emotional insight, and contextual relevance, as reflected in outcome-based evaluations (Chew, Maniam, and Sim, 2024), scalable assessment systems (Gervasi, Müller, and Reiter, 2022), and research on emotional well-being (Hatamnejad, Farhadi, and Zarei, 2023). This shift challenges classical rationality, as Nie, Zhang, and Lie (2021) show through behavioural inconsistency in public health compliance, and highlights the need to integrate psychosocial nuance with epidemiological reasoning, as argued by Lazzari and Rabottini (2025a; 2025b). Taken together, these insights position pandemics as catalysts that redefine ethical priorities, reconfigure the nature of educational and social reality, and transform the epistemic conditions under which knowledge is produced, shared, and enacted (Table 9).

Table 9: Summative table

Concept	Explanation	Application
Axiology:	Analyses values and ethics, particularly how crises such as pandemics reshape societal priorities—highlighting the importance of solidarity, emotional resilience, and adaptability.	Axiology informs the integration of interprofessional education (IPE) into national curricula (Kaap-Fröhlich, Müller, and Reimann, 2022). It supports reflective mobile learning as an ethical means of promoting well-being (Hatamnejad, Farhadi, and Zarei, 2023).
Ontology:	Regarding the nature of being and existence, pandemics disrupt assumptions about learning and social interaction, revealing them to be embodied, situated, and relational.	Ontology validates the EMeA model as a dynamic educational process (Chew, Maniam, and Sim, 2024); supports decentralised digital assessment (Gervasi, Müller, and Reiter, 2022); and aligns with ontological stratification (Guerrero Fernandez, 2022).
Epistemology:	Explores how knowledge is created, validated, and shared; pandemic conditions challenge fixed institutional models and highlight emotional, contextual, and diverse ways of knowing.	Epistemology operationalises knowledge through real-time, experience-sensitive evaluations (Chew, Maniam, and Sim, 2024); it supports emotionally attuned infrastructures (Gervasi, Müller, and Reiter, 2022) and addresses behavioural inconsistency in public health (Nie, Zhang, and Li, 2021).

CHAPTER 7

Conclusions and the Phenomenology of Pandemics

Introduction to health behaviours during pandemics

The concepts of pathophilia and Samos Syndrome, developed through a series of publications by Lazzari and Rabottini (2022b; 2024a; 2024b), offer a transdisciplinary framework for understanding behavioural resistance to contagion during pandemics. Rather than treating non-compliance with public health measures as irrational or incidental, the authors argue that specific psychological profiles—particularly those involving borderline personality disorder (BPD), trauma histories, and pathophilic tendencies—actively engage with illness as a form of existential expression.

In their foundational paper, Lazzari and Rabottini (2022b) argue that pandemics persist not only through biological transmission but also through deep-rooted psychological and phenomenological dynamics. They introduce Samos Syndrome as a behavioural pattern in which individuals, often with BPD, reject protective behaviours and instead engage with illness through symbolic, relational, or self-harming mechanisms. These behaviours challenge conventional epidemiological models that assume a universal motivation to preserve health.

Building on this, Lazzari (2023a; 2023b) examines the specific vulnerabilities of individuals with personality disorders during pandemics, emphasising increased risks of sexually transmitted infections and HIV. The study links these risks to emotional instability, trauma, and a form of pathophilia—where illness serves as a medium for identity development and emotional regulation. The author contends that these behaviours are not merely maladaptive but reflect a deeper engagement with contagion as a relational and existential phenomenon.

The last two publications (Lazzari and Rabottini, 2024a; 2024b), published in the journal *European Psychiatry*, strengthen the syndrome's theoretical and epidemiological implications. They propose that Samos Syndrome explains why transmissible diseases persist despite widespread awareness and prevention efforts. The syndrome is redefined as a phenomenological structure—a way of being-in-the-world in which contagion is sometimes accepted rather than avoided. This enigmatic conclusion enables a more detailed understanding of how pandemics spread, particularly among marginalised groups with complex psychological profiles. Together, these works position Samos Syndrome as a conceptual bridge uniting psychological, ethical, and existential aspects of pandemic behaviour. It challenges the idea that all individuals pursue health and safety, revealing how some may engage with contagion for personal, relational, or symbolic reasons. This framework has implications for public health strategies, clinical interventions, and ethical debates, particularly when addressing populations whose behavioural responses to illness contradict traditional, rational and relational models of knowledge production and sharing (Lazzari, 1992).

Psychological depth and irrationalism

The concept of Samos Syndrome, developed by Lazzari and Rabottini (2022b; 2024a; 2024b), offers a transdisciplinary framework for understanding pandemic-related behaviours that challenge conventional public health logic. Rather than treating non-compliance as irrational or rebellious, the syndrome reinterprets these behaviours as psychologically, ethically, and phenomenologically meaningful responses to contagion. This model integrates clinical psychiatry, trauma theory, and existential inquiry, providing a coherent perspective on symbolic, compulsive, and ethically charged actions.

At its core, Samos Syndrome describes the psychological depth and irrationality that characterise certain behaviours during a pandemic—such as pathophilia, denial, and parasuicidal risk-taking. These actions are not random but reflect unconscious drives and emotional dysregulation, particularly among individuals diagnosed with borderline personality disorder (BPD). Lazzari and Rabottini (2022b) propose that these patterns stem from trauma histories and relational instability, creating a behavioural framework shaped by fear, symbolic meaning, and existential disorientation. In a subsequent study, Lazzari (2023a; 2023b) shows that people with BPD engage in high-risk sexual behaviours during pandemics not out of ignorance but as methods of identity repair and emotional regulation. These findings resonate with broader debates on irrationalism, in which unconscious motives and symbolic acts of control and surrender drive pandemic behaviours.

Beyond its psychological aspect, Samos Syndrome highlights the phenomenological experience of contagion. Public health behaviours—such as masking, distancing, and isolation—are not seen as neutral mandates but as emotionally and symbolically significant rituals. Lazzari and Rabottini (2024) examine how individuals with BPD engage with these behaviours from a trauma-informed perspective, showing how relational instability and pathophilic tendencies shape their embodied responses to risk. This perspective aligns with phenomenological insights from Butler (2022), Ritunnano and colleagues (2023), and Lazzari and Rabottini (2025a; 2025b), all of which emphasise the importance of public health behaviours within lived narratives and moral frameworks.

The ethical implications of Samos Syndrome are equally significant. Pandemic behaviour is reinterpreted as ethically meaningful, with each action—or omission—constituting a gesture of harm or care. Lazzari and Rabottini (2024a; 2024b) show that emotionally driven decision-making among people with BPD heightens transmission risks while also serving as a search for intimacy, validation, and coherence. This redefinition shifts the ethical debate from a sole focus on individual rights to one that recognises shared obligations and relational accountability. In this context, moral agency is shaped by vulnerability, trauma, and the pursuit of ontological stability.

Furthermore, Samos Syndrome emphasises the existential dimensions of pandemic behaviour. Risk-taking appears to strengthen emotional bonds and serves as a symbolic act of devotion, resistance, or identity reaffirmation. Lazzari's early research on HIV/AIDS patients (1992) laid the groundwork for understanding how vulnerability and biological risk trigger significant psychological and ethical shifts. In his 2023 study, Lazzari shows that people with BPD and trauma histories engage in high-risk sexual behaviour during pandemics as expressions of existential longing and relational healing. These findings reveal how intimacy and contagion are often intertwined in the search for meaning, and how pandemic behaviour—although potentially harmful—can reflect deeply human efforts to reclaim agency and connection.

Taken together, these insights position Samos Syndrome as a conceptual bridge linking psychological vulnerability, ethical complexity, and phenomenological depth. The framework challenges traditional assumptions about health-seeking behaviour and promotes a more nuanced, interdisciplinary approach to behavioural epidemiology. By integrating clinical psychiatry with public health and social theory, Samos Syndrome offers a robust model for understanding how trauma, symbolic meaning, and relational instability shape human responses to contagion.

The concept of Samos Syndrome, developed by Lazzari and collaborators (Lazzari and Rabottini, 2022a; 2022b; 2024a; 2024b; 2025a; 2025b), offers a multidimensional framework for interpreting pandemic behaviour that extends beyond the limits of epidemiological modelling or rational choice theory. Rather than reducing public health non-compliance to ignorance or defiance, the framework views pandemic behaviour as a complex interplay of psychological drives, ethical tensions, and existential meaning-making. By integrating clinical psychiatry, trauma theory, and phenomenological inquiry, Samos Syndrome provides a cohesive perspective for understanding symbolic, compulsive, and ethically charged actions.

At its core, the syndrome involves irrational, emotionally charged behaviours—such as pathophilia, denial, and parasuicidal risk-taking—that emerge during pandemics. These actions are not random but reflect unconscious drives and emotional dysregulation, particularly among individuals diagnosed with borderline personality disorder (BPD). Lazzari and Rabottini (2022a; 2022b) argue that such patterns stem from trauma histories and relational instability, forming a behavioural framework shaped by fear, symbolic meaning, and existential disorientation. In a later study, Lazzari (2023a; 2023b) shows that persons with BPD engage in high-risk sexual behaviours during pandemics not as acts of ignorance but as strategies for identity repair and emotional regulation. These findings contribute to broader discussions of irrationalism, in which unconscious motives and symbolic acts of control and surrender drive pandemic behaviour.

Beyond its psychological depth, Samos Syndrome highlights the phenomenological experience of contagion. Public health behaviours—such as masking, distancing, and isolation—are not merely neutral mandates but emotionally and symbolically significant rituals. Lazzari and Rabottini (2024a; 2025a; 2025b) examine how individuals with BPD engage with these behaviours from a trauma-informed perspective, showing how relational instability and pathophilic tendencies shape their embodied responses to risk. This interpretation aligns with contemporary phenomenological scholarship, including Butler (2022), Ritunnano and colleagues (2023), and Drożdżowicz (2020), all of whom emphasise the embeddedness of public health behaviours within lived narratives and moral frameworks. In cognitive science, this approach also guides the integration of first-person perspectives with empirical models, thereby enhancing understanding of perception and consciousness (Fernandez and Doyon, 2025).

A recent phenomenological essay by Lazzari and Rabottini (2025a; 2025b) further examines the subjective and emotional dimensions of individuals' experiences during public health crises. Rather than emphasising empirical metrics or clinical outcomes, this perspective focuses on how people perceive, interpret, and emotionally engage with preventive mandates. Mask-wearing, for instance, may evoke feelings of protection, exclusion, or solidarity, depending on social and cultural contexts. Likewise, isolation may provide a sense of safety from contagion while also causing loneliness or existential unease (Ritunnano et al., 2023). A phenomenological perspective captures these affective and interpretive layers, showing how individuals incorporate public health behaviours into their moral frameworks and personal stories. Lockdown conditions often distort temporal perceptions, transforming public spaces into symbols of threat or yearning. Butler (2022) describes this disruption as a reorientation of everyday meaning and relationality, fostering reflection on shared vulnerability and interdependence.

The ethical implications of Samos Syndrome are equally important. Pandemic behaviour is ethically significant, with each action—or omission—constituting a gesture of harm or care. Lazzari and Rabottini (2024a) show that emotionally driven decision-making among persons with BPD increases transmission risks while also serving as a search for intimacy, validation, and coherence. This redefinition shifts the ethical debate from a focus on individual rights to recognition of shared obligations and relational accountability. Moral agency, in this context, is influenced by vulnerability, trauma, and the need for ontological stability.

Samos Syndrome also draws attention to the existential forces that shape human behaviour during pandemics. Risk-taking can deepen emotional bonds and serve as a symbolic expression of loyalty, defiance, or an attempt to restore a threatened sense of identity. Lazzari's early work with individuals living with HIV/AIDS (1992) demonstrated how experiences of vulnerability and biological risk can prompt profound psychological and ethical transformations. Building on this foundation, his 2023 study shows that people with borderline personality disorder and trauma histories may engage in high-risk sexual behaviour during pandemics as a form of existential longing and an effort to repair or reaffirm relationships. Together, these findings reveal how intimacy and contagion can become intertwined in the search for meaning, and how pandemic-related behaviours—despite their potential harm—often reflect deeply human attempts to reclaim agency, connection, and emotional coherence.

Using Samos Syndrome as an integrative concept allows pandemic health behaviours to be understood as emotionally intelligent, ethically grounded, and phenomenologically rich. This approach synthesises diverse disciplinary sources and offers a new contribution to public health scholarship: a theory of pandemic behaviour centred on psychological vulnerability, embodied experience, and relational ethics. It challenges normative ideas about health-seeking behaviour and advocates a more nuanced, interdisciplinary understanding of how people navigate contagion, community, and care during crises.

Structural aspects: What pandemics are

We redefine pandemics as psychosocial and existential events rather than merely biological outbreaks. We have described pandemics as sometimes triggered by unconscious drives, particularly pathophilia, a compulsive attraction to risk and contagion, suggesting that unexpected, impulsive health behaviours that clash with primary prevention campaigns help create conditions for viral spread. This central idea is further developed in our later studies, which portray pandemics as identity-driven crises characterised by impulsiveness, emotional fragmentation, solipsism, and symbolic acts of vulnerability. These dynamics align with phenomenological psychiatry, which emphasises relational instability and subjective disruption.

A pandemic is regarded not only as a biological threat but also as an ontological rupture that transforms individuals' sense of being-in-the-world. Cases of pandemic-related psychosis, such as attempted suicide to escape Covid-19 threats, documented in our clinical literature, illustrate how existential fear can fracture identity, distort perceptions of reality, and destabilise relational meaning. These episodes suggest the emergence of irrationalism—not merely a cognitive error but a worldview rooted in emotion, instinct, and symbolic belief. During pandemics, irrationalism becomes particularly prominent, as psychological stress and existential threats overshadow practical logic. At other times, personal experience transforms an apparent irrationalism not into a knowledge failure but into a conscious existential choice, that is, one that rejects official health behaviours and frameworks and embraces alterative meanings to objectivist world views; for example, alternative and holistic therapies might challenge current scientific knowledge and therapies in infection control and vaccination campaigns.

Our research on HIV-related behaviours further develops this perspective through the lens of Samos Syndrome, in which individuals knowingly expose themselves to transmissible diseases as parasuicidal or symbolic acts. In these cases, irrationality is not a failure of knowledge but a conscious existential stance—one that challenges normative health behaviours and embraces risk as a means of creating meaning. In times of a viral pandemic, individuals become potential vectors of harm or care, and everyday choices—such as attending gatherings, skipping preventive measures, or refusing to wear masks—are no longer private decisions but ethically and socially charged acts. These actions influence the health outcomes of vulnerable populations and the resilience of public systems. The moral landscape shifts from individual rights to shared responsibilities, requiring a re-evaluation of civic duty, ethical agency, and social solidarity. A pandemic reveals a layered ontology of responsibility, in which individuals are part of networks of interdependence and where both actions and omissions have social, psychological, and institutional repercussions.

This interconnected framework has significant implications for public health and pandemic management. It emphasises that effective response strategies must integrate ethical reasoning with scientific and policy decisions, draw on diverse evidence, including behavioural and narrative insights, address emotional and relational challenges in health communication, account for identity-driven behaviour and personal experiences in preventive measures, and prioritise ethical engagement and relational care in public health interventions. Overall, these perspectives promote a human-centred, psychologically aware, and ethically sensitive approach to public health—one that recognises the emotional, symbolic, and relational aspects of pandemic behaviour and integrates them into prevention, communication, and care strategies.

Policies and future directions in pandemic prevention

The behavioural and existential dynamics identified in our research on pandemics call for a shift in public health policy—one that integrates psychological understanding, ethical considerations, and real-time behavioural data. Psychosocial screening should be incorporated into pandemic response protocols to identify individuals at increased risk of pathophilic behaviours. Trauma-informed assessments must be tailored to detect emotional dysregulation, relational instability, and symbolic engagement with contagion, particularly among populations with emotional friability or histories of interpersonal trauma. These screenings would enable early identification of behavioural vulnerabilities that could undermine containment efforts.

Targeted education should go beyond basic health messages to address the emotional and symbolic reasons for rejecting health behaviours. Culturally sensitive campaigns should be tailored to different psychological profiles, recognising fear, identity fragmentation, and relational longing as drivers of non-compliance. Such messaging would foster emotional literacy and relational awareness in public discourse. Ethical triage models are essential for supporting morally grounded decision-making, particularly during psychiatric admissions in crises. Predictive tools should be developed to balance compassion with resource allocation, recognising the complexity of behavioural risk and the relational needs of vulnerable individuals. Principles of fairness, dignity, and contextual awareness must guide these models.

Digital monitoring enables the detection of emerging behavioural trends and supports real-time interventions. Web-based ethnographic platforms and behavioural analytics can identify groups exhibiting symbolic risk-taking, emotional distress, and relational disruption. These tools support adaptable communication and enable responsive governance aligned with evolving psychological landscapes. Together, these policy directions emphasise the need to integrate psychological depth, ethical nuance, and phenomenological awareness into pandemic preparedness and response. By recognising the emotional, symbolic, and relational aspects of contagion, public health strategy can become more inclusive and resilient—one that values the complexity of human behaviour under existential threat.

Conclusions

Our research on pandemics offers a conceptual framework for understanding pandemic-related behaviours across the intersecting fields of psychology, ethics, and phenomenology. As outlined in our studies, irrational, impulsive, and emotionally intense reactions can occur during periods of contagion, particularly among individuals with emotional frailty and those who rely on solipsistic knowledge. These behaviours—such as pathophilic tendencies and parasuicidal risk-taking—are not merely clinical anomalies; they reflect more profound existential confusion and symbolic interactions with risk

(Lazzari, 2023a; 2023b). By emphasising the lived experience of public health mandates and the embodied meaning of pandemic rituals, we have proposed models of pandemic preparedness that integrate phenomenological insight with social theory, creating a framework that is both diagnostically and conceptually comprehensive.

As Lazzari and Rabottini (2024a; 2024b) note, pandemic-related actions are not ethically neutral; they are relational gestures shaped by trauma, civic duty, and ontological vulnerability. We should reinterpret intimacy and contagion as interconnected forces, in which high-risk behaviours may serve as acts of devotion, identity reclamation, or existential affirmation (Lazzari, 1992; 2023a; 2023b). This view calls for a shift in public health ethics—from individualised behavioural compliance to relational models of care, solidarity, and accountability. In this way, we aim to foster a deeper understanding of pandemic psychology and broaden the moral vocabulary for interpreting, contextualising, and addressing such behaviours.

During the Covid-19 lockdown in the United Kingdom, young adults faced a deep tension between public health guidelines and their personal need for intimacy. Research by Owens and colleagues (2021) shows that sexual desire did not simply fade under the weight of rational knowledge about contagion; instead, it changed form. Solo sexual activity increased as individuals sought private outlets, while partnered activity decreased because of contact restrictions. Within relationships, confinement produced mixed outcomes: for some couples, bonds were strained, and satisfaction decreased, while others reported feeling closer and experiencing renewed intimacy.

This study highlights the gap between propositional knowledge and lived conviction. Participants recognised the risks of close contact during a pandemic, yet emotional imperatives—connection, stress relief, and the assertion of will—often outweighed rational adherence to prevention campaigns. In this way, Owens and colleagues (2021) highlight the same philosophical divide evident in the book's concepts: the prioritisation of intuition, emotion, and subjective immediacy over collective rationality. Public health messaging, grounded in universality and evidence, clashed with the sovereignty of personal belief and desire, demonstrating that resistance to prevention is not merely ignorance but a structural aspect of human behaviour in crisis.

In ongoing debates about pandemic prevention, Professor Yitka Graham's work highlights the challenges of securing public adherence to health campaigns. In a study of bariatric surgery patients, Graham and colleagues examined how individuals responded to the requirement for lifelong micronutrient supplementation, a preventive measure intended to reduce the risk of serious complications (Mahawar et al., 2019). The findings showed that although patients recognised the rational necessity of supplementation, many struggled to adhere consistently. Emotional responses, daily routines, and personal interpretations often outweighed the abstract knowledge of medical risk.

This narrative directly relates to the broader issue of pandemic prevention. Just as bariatric patients resist supplementation despite understanding its importance, populations during pandemics often resist public health measures such as vaccination, social distancing, or mask-wearing. The gap between propositional knowledge—knowing what science recommends—and lived conviction—believing what feels immediate or manageable—becomes the fault line where prevention fails. Graham's work emphasises that resistance is not merely ignorance but a structural aspect of human behaviour: individuals interpret health advice through emotion, intuition, and personal experience.

During the global rollout of Covid-19 vaccines, Raw, Rees, Kelly, Wroe, and Chadwick (2022) examined how prior infection affected the occurrence of adverse events following vaccination with popular vaccines. They found that individuals who had previously contracted Covid-19 were more likely to report adverse events after the first dose, but this association did not persist after the second dose. The results suggest that immunological memory from natural infection may heighten the body's initial response to vaccination, leading to more severe side effects. In contrast, subsequent doses more closely align with the experiences of the general population.

This research highlights the tension between scientific knowledge and personal responses, including biological ones. Public health campaigns emphasise the safety and need for vaccination, yet individuals often interpret their experiences through the lens of lived reality. For those with prior infection, heightened adverse events after the first dose of a vaccine may reinforce scepticism or hesitation, even when evidence supports continued vaccination. The study by Raw and colleagues (2022) shows that knowing that vaccines are safe and effective does not always lead to belief or acceptance of this truth when personal experience suggests otherwise.

In the context of pandemic prevention, this insight is crucial. Campaigns that rely solely on rational persuasion often conflict with individuals' personal beliefs and experiences (e.g., adverse vaccine reactions), leading to interpretive differences and resistance. Professor Graham's research shows that prevention must consider the ontological basis of lived conviction, where truth is more influenced by what is felt and experienced than by evidence. This view aligns with our pandemic framework, in which intuition and emotion often replace reason, making it sometimes difficult for prevention campaigns to achieve compliance.

References

AdoleScienza.it (2025). 'Sindrome di Samo e il desiderio di contrarre malattie'. Available from: https://www.adolescienza.it/sessualita-amori-amicizie/sindrome-di-samo-ed-il-desiderio-di-contrarre-malattie

Ahmad, A.R., and Murad, H.R. (2020). 'The impact of social media on panic during the COVID19 pandemic in Iraqi Kurdistan: online questionnaire study', *Journal of Medical Internet Research*, 22(5), e19556.

Alam, S., Choudhury, T., and Rahman, M. (2023). 'Do social media influencers influence the vaccination drive?', *International Journal of Forecasting*, 39(1), pp. 88–102. Available from: https://www.sciencedirect.com/science/study/pii/S0169207023000123

Alsharji, K.E. (2022). 'Anxiety and depression during the COVID19 pandemic in Kuwait: the role of coping strategies', *Psychology Research and Behavior Management*, 15, pp. 283–294.

Babicki, M., Szewczykowska, I., and MastalerzMigas, A. (2021). 'Mental health in the era of COVID19: prevalence of depression, anxiety and insomnia in a Polish population', *International Journal of Environmental Research and Public Health*, 18(23), 11862.

Barton, D.A., Lee, R., and Cacioppo, S. (2023). 'A translational neuroscience perspective on loneliness', *Neuroscience and Biobehavioral Reviews*, 143(1), pp. 104–117. Available from: https://www.sciencedirect.com/science/study/pii/S0149763423000456

Batteux, E., Taylor, A., and Carter, H. (2021). *The Impact of the COVID-19 Pandemic on Adult Mental Health in the UK: A Rapid Systematic Review*. Public Health England, UK. Available from: https://www.gov.uk/government/publications/impact-of-Covid-19-on-adult-mental-health

Beauchamp, T.L., and Childress, J.F. (2013). *Principles of Biomedical Ethics*. 7th edn. New York: Oxford University Press.

Becerra, M.B., Becerra, B.J., and Tejada, S. (2021). 'COVID19 and mental health: the impact of the pandemic on Latinos in the U.S.', *Journal of Racial and Ethnic Health Disparities*, 8, pp. 1546–1552.

Bell, K. (2018). 'The "problem" of undesigned relationality: Ethnographic fieldwork, dual roles and research ethics', *Ethnography*, 20(1), pp. 8–26.

Bell, K., and Green, J. (2022). 'On the limits of behavioural public health: Rethinking risk, responsibility and pandemic response', *Critical Public Health*, 32(5), pp. 657–669.

Birks, M., and Mills, J. (2015). *Grounded Theory: A Practical Guide*. 2nd edn. London: Sage Publications.

Borlotti, G. (2015). *Irrationalism and the Limits of Reason*. University of Birmingham Lecture Series.

Brenner, C. (1988). *An Elementary Textbook of Psychoanalysis*. New York: Anchor Books.

Broadbent, A. (2013). *Philosophy of Epidemiology*. London: Palgrave Macmillan.

Broadbent, A. (2020). *Philosophy of Epidemiology*. Cambridge: Cambridge University Press.

Broadbent, A. (2022). 'Philosophy of medicine and COVID-19: must do better', *Philosophy of Medicine*, 3(1), pp. 1–6.

Bryant, A., and Charmaz, K. (2007). *The SAGE Handbook of Grounded Theory*. London: Sage Publications.

Butler, J. (2022). *What World Is This? A Pandemic Phenomenology*. New York: Columbia University Press.

Cambridge Dictionary (2024a). 'Irrationality'. Available from: https://dictionary.cambridge.org

Cambridge Dictionary (2024b). 'Rationality'. [online] Available from: https://dictionary.cambridge.org

Cambridge Dictionary (2025a). 'Pandemic'. Available from: https://dictionary.cambridge.org/dictionary/english/pandemic

Cambridge Dictionary (2025b). 'Rationality'. Cambridge: Cambridge University Press. Available from: https://dictionary.cambridge.org/dictionary/english/rationality

Canpolat, C., and Yildirim, M. (2021). 'Meaning in life, psychological flexibility, and psychological symptoms during the COVID19 pandemic', *Journal of Clinical Psychology*, 77(8), pp. 1865–1878.

Caperon, L., Saville, F., and Ahern, S. (2022). 'Developing a socio-ecological model for community engagement in a health programme in an under-served urban area', PLOS ONE, 17(9), e0275092.

Carel, H. (2018). 'Illness as a phenomenological challenge'. In: M. Solomon, J.R. Simon, and H. Kincaid (eds.), *The Routledge Companion to Philosophy of Medicine*. London: Routledge, pp. 247–256.

Carel, H. (2020). 'Masking the self: Embodiment and disruption in pandemic life', *Journal of Medical Humanities*, 41(3), pp. 245–260.

Carter, S.M., and Little, M. (2007). 'Justifying knowledge, justifying method, taking action: Epistemologies, methodologies, and methods in qualitative research', *Qualitative Health Research*, 17(10), pp. 1316–1328.

CDC (Centers for Disease Control and Prevention) (2024). *NERD Academy: What Exactly Is a Pandemic*? Available from: https://www.cdc.gov/nerd-academy/defining-a-pandemic/index.html

Celbis, O., Van de Laar, M., and Volante, L. (2023). *Resilience in Higher Education Settings During the COVID-19 Pandemic: A Scoping Literature Review with Implications for Policy and Practice*. Maastricht University. [online] Available from: https://cris.maastrichtuniversity.nl/en/publications/resilience-in-higher-education-settings-during-the-covid-19-pande/

Ceronetti, G. (1993). *The Silence of the Body: Materials for the Study of Medicine*. New York: Farrar, Straus and Giroux.

Chew, L., Tan, R., and Ong, S. (2024). 'Interprofessional education in mental health: A scoping review', *Journal of Interprofessional Care*, 38(1), pp. 45–60.

Chew, Q.H., Maniam, E.J.H., and Sim, K. (2024). 'Inter-Professional Education Interventions, and Practice Outcomes Related to Healthcare Setting and Patients within Mental Healthcare: A Scoping Review', *Perspectives on Medical Education*, 13(1), pp. 108–118.

Churchill, S.D. (2014). 'Phenomenology'. In: T. Teo (ed.), *Encyclopedia of Critical Psychology*. New York: Springer, pp. 1389–1402.

Claus, M., De Backer, J., Van den Eede, F., Vanderhasselt, M.A., and De Raedt, R. (2022). 'Longterm psychiatric sequelae of COVID19 ICU admission: a prospective cohort study', *Journal of Critical Care*, 70, 154070.

Cohen, L., Manion, L., and Morrison, K. (2018). *Research Methods in Education*. 8th edn. London: Routledge.

Collins English Dictionary (2024). 'Irrationalism'. [online] Available from: https://www.collinsdictionary.com

Corbett, A., Ballard, C., and PROTECT Study Group (2022). 'Cognitive decline in older adults in the UK during and after the COVID-19 pandemic', *Age and Ageing*, 51(6), pp. 1–9.

Crawford, J. (2023). 'COVID-19 and higher education: A pandemic response model from rapid adaptation to consolidation and restoration'. *The International Education Journal: Comparative Perspectives*, 22(1).

Creswell, J.W., and Poth, C.N. (2018). *Qualitative Inquiry and Research Design: Choosing Among Five Approaches*. 4th edn. Thousand Oaks, CA: SAGE Publications.

Crotty, M. (1998). *The Foundations of Social Research: Meaning and Perspective in the Research Process*. London: SAGE Publications.

de Lima, M.G. (2020). *Os aspectos existenciais do sofrimento humano: uma abordagem fenomenológica no cuidado em saúde*. Fortaleza: Universidade Federal do Ceará.

Dewey, J. (1925). *Experience and Nature*. Chicago: Open Court.

Dewey, J. (1927). *The Public and its Problems*. Athens: Ohio University Press.

Dewey, J. (1939). *Freedom and Culture*. New York: Putnam.

Dictionary Online (2024). 'Irrationalism'. Oakland: Dictionary.com, LLC. Available from: https://www.dictionary.com

Dongol, Y., Maharjan, R., Shrestha, A., Shrestha, S., and Shrestha, R. (2022). 'Impact of COVID19 on sleep quality and stress among university students: a crosssectional study', *PLOS ONE*, 17(4), e0266976.

Douglas, H. (2009). *Science, Policy, and the Value-Free Ideal*. Pittsburgh: University of Pittsburgh Press.

Drożdżowicz, A. (2020). 'Increasing the Role of Phenomenology in Psychiatric Diagnosis–The Clinical Staging Approach', *Journal of Medicine and Philosophy*, 45(6), pp. 683–702.

Duman, N. (2021). 'Psychological resilience, depression, anxiety, and stress during the COVID19 pandemic in Turkey', *Psychology, Health & Medicine*, 27(2), pp. 304–316.

Dupré, J., and Leonelli, S. (2022). 'Process epistemology in the COVID-19 era: rethinking the research process to avoid dangerous forms of reification', *European Journal for Philosophy of Science*, 12(20).

Durkheim, É. (1991). *Suicide: A Study in Sociology*. Translated by J.A. Spaulding and G. Simpson. London: Routledge. (Originally published in 1897.)

Encyclopaedia Britannica (2024a). 'Irrationalism'. London: Encyclopaedia Britannica, Inc. Available from: https://www.britannica.com/ [Accessed: 30 October 2025].

Encyclopaedia Britannica (2024b). 'Solipsism'. London: Encyclopaedia Britannica, Inc. Available from: https://www.britannica.com/topic/solipsism [Accessed: 30 October 2025].

Erciyes, E. (2019). *Three Pillars of Phenomenology: Husserl, Heidegger and Merleau-Ponty*. Memphis: University of Memphis Philosophy Department.

Erjavac, M., Volavšek, M., Štefančič, M., and Dernovšek, M.Z. (2023). 'Acute child and adolescent psychiatric emergencies during the COVID19 pandemic: a retrospective observational study', *Frontiers in Psychiatry*, 14, 1123451.

Fancourt, D., Steptoe, A., and Bu, F. (2021). 'Trajectories of anxiety and depressive symptoms during enforced isolation due to COVID19 in England: a longitudinal observational study', *The Lancet Psychiatry*, 8(2), pp. 141–149.

Fernandez, A.V., and Doyon, M. (2025). 'Phenomenology and the Cognitive Sciences', *Phenomenology and the Cognitive Sciences*, 24(4).

Finlay, L. (2009), 'Debating phenomenological research methods', *Phenomenology and Practice*, 3(1), pp. 6–25.

Flick, U. (2018). *An Introduction to Qualitative Research*. 6th edn. London: SAGE Publications.

Freud, A. (1936). *The Ego and the Mechanisms of Defence*. London: Hogarth Press and Institute of Psycho-Analysis.

Freud, S. (1901). *The Psychopathology of Everyday Life*. Translated by A.A. Brill. New York: Macmillan.

Gervasi, L., Müller, T., and Reiter, S. (2022). 'Secure electronic written exams in medical education: Lessons from the pandemic', *Medical Education Technology*, 18(2), pp. 112–124.

Gervasi, O., Perri, D., and Simonetti, M. (2022). 'Strategies and system implementations for secure electronic written exams', *IEEE Access*, 10, pp. 20559–20570. doi: 10.1109/ACCESS.2022.3150860.

Glaser, B.G., and Strauss, A.L. (1967). *The Discovery of Grounded Theory: Strategies for Qualitative Research*. Chicago: Aldine Publishing.

GMC (General Medical Council) (2024). *Decision Making and Consent*. London: GMC. https://www.gmc-uk.org/cdn/documents/gmc-guidance-for-doctors---decision-making-and-consent-english_pdf-84191055.pdf

Goedert, J.J., Pizza, G., Gritti, F.M., Costigliola, P., Boschini, A., Bini, A., Lazzari, C., and Palareti, A. (1995). 'Mortality among drug users in the AIDS era', *International Journal of Epidemiology*, 24(6), pp. 1204–1210.

Green, J., and Thorogood, N. (2018). *Qualitative Methods for Health Research*. 4th edn. London: Sage Publications.

Grix, J. (2010). *The Foundations of Research*. 2nd edn. London: Palgrave Macmillan.

Guarnera, J., Yuen, E., and Macpherson, H. (2023). 'The impact of loneliness and social isolation on cognitive ageing: A narrative review', *Journal of Alzheimer's Disease*, 95(2).

Guba, E.G., and Lincoln, Y.S. (1994). 'Competing paradigms in qualitative research', in Denzin, N.K., and Lincoln, Y.S. (eds.), *Handbook of Qualitative Research*. Thousand Oaks, CA: Sage, pp. 105–117.

Guerrero Fernandez, A. (2022). 'Ontological stratification and the layered nature of pandemics', *Journal of Philosophy and Health*, 14(3), pp. 211–228.

Guzman, V., Doyle, F., Foley, R., et al. (2023). 'Socio-ecological determinants of older people's mental health and well-being during COVID-19', *Frontiers in Public Health*, 11, p. 1148758.

Hanna, K.L., Smith, J., and Thomas, R. (2023). 'The association between loneliness or social isolation and food and eating behaviours: A scoping review', *Public Health Nutrition*, 26(4), pp. 512–528.

Hatamnejad, M., Farhadi, A., and Zarei, S. (2023). 'Emotional intelligence and happiness among clinical students during COVID-19', *Journal of Medical Psychology*, 29(3), pp. 201–215.

Husserl, E. (1931). *Ideas: General Introduction to Pure Phenomenology.* London: George Allen and Unwin.

Iglesias-Pradas, S., Hernández-García, Á., Chaparro-Peláez, J., and Prieto, J.L. (2021). 'Emergency remote teaching and students' academic performance in higher education during the COVID-19 pandemic: A case study'. *Computers in Human Behavior*, 119, 106713.

Jatobá, A., Castro-Nunes, P., and Rodrigues de Carvalho, P.V. (2025). 'On the epistemology of resilience in public health: a novel perspective in a changing world', *Frontiers in Health Services*, 4, 1453006.

Jukić, V., Jakovljević, M., Šagud, M., Lončar, M., Crnković, D., VuksanĆusa, B., Janović, Š., and Pivac, N. (2020). 'First admission of a patient with pandemicinduced psychosis', *Psychiatria Danubina*, 32(3), pp. 345–348.

Jumaa, J.A., Catena, R., Brown, E., Sanyang, S., Tridico, A., and Weaver, D. (2023). 'Exploring pandemic preparedness in higher education: Lessons learnt from students' lived experiences during a critical time', *Discover Health Systems*, 2, p. 9.

Kaap-Fröhlich, S., Müller, C., and Reimann, P. (2022). 'Position paper on interprofessional education in German-speaking countries', *GMS Journal for Medical Education*, 39(4), Doc45.

Kang, H., Yamamoto, T., and Saito, Y. (2023). 'Nurses' perception towards care robots during COVID-19', *Geriatric Nursing*, 44(2), pp. 78–85.

Kaplan, D.M. (1989). *The Psychodynamics of Altruistic Surrender.* New York: Basic Books.

Khan, K.S., Mamun, M.A., Griffiths, M.D., and Ullah, I. (2021). 'The mental health impact of the COVID19 pandemic across different cohorts: a systematic review', *International Journal of Mental Health and Addiction*, 19, pp. 1–27.

Koca, F. (2022). 'COVID-19 outbreak: Mitigating role of college students' emotional intelligence in the relationship between psychological distress and academic satisfaction', *Psychiatria Danubina*, 34(1), pp. 133–140.

Krieger, N. (2020). 'Measures of exposure and risk: Understanding the social patterning of COVID-19', *American Journal of Public Health*, 110(7), pp. 935–936.

La Rosa Nera (2022). *Sindrome di Samo: l'amore ignoto per la malattia*. Available from: https://www.larosanera.it/sindrome-di-samo-l%e2%80%99amore-ignoto-per-la-malattia

Larki, M., Bahri, N., Moghri, J., and Latifnejad Roudsari, R. (202). 'Living with Discordance: A Qualitative Description of the Challenges Faced by HIV Negative Married Women', *Int J Community Based Nurs Midwifery*, 8(2), pp. 103–115. doi: 10.30476/IJCBNM.2020.82845.1093. PMID: 32309452; PMCID: PMC7153425.

Lawson, T. (2012). 'Ontology and the study of social reality: emergence, organisation, community, power, social relations, corporations, artefacts and money', *Cambridge Journal of Economics*, 36(2), pp. 345–385.

Lazzari, C. (1992). *Guida all'assistenza psicologica del paziente HIV positivo e con AIDS* [Guide to the psychological care of HIV-positive and AIDS patients]. Bologna: Pàtron Editore.

Lazzari, C. (2012). 'La Sindrome di Samo' [Samos syndrome], *Rivista di Sessuologia Clinica*. Milan: FrancoAngeli.

Lazzari, C. (2020). 'Psychiatry during COVID-19 pandemic: A case report of attempted mercy killing', *Psychiatria Danubina*, 32(2), pp. 303–304.

Lazzari, C. (2023a). 'Samos Syndrome, persons with borderline personality disorder and risk for sexually transmitted infections and HIV: Their role during pandemics', *Current Innovations in Disease and Health Research*, 7, pp. 12–21.

Lazzari, C. (2023b). 'Persons with borderline personality disorder and pathophilia: understanding causes of pandemic diffusion of transmissible diseases through Samos Syndrome', *European Psychiatry*. Cambridge University Press. Available from: https://www.cambridge.org/core/journals/european-psychiatry/study/persons-with-borderline-personality-disorder-and-pathophilia-understanding-causes-of-pandemic-diffusion-of-transmissible-diseases-through-samos-syndrome/831C4BA8ACA3E094B1C82E78F9121434 [Accessed: 8 July 2025].

Lazzari, C., Colleoni, G.G., and Trallo, F. (1995). *Ninfee alla deriva. Aspetti psicosociali dell'AIDS e delle altre malattie a trasmissione sessuale* [Water lilies adrift: psychosocial aspects of AIDS and other sexually transmitted diseases]. Bologna: Pitagora Editrice. Available from: Unilibro.

Lazzari, C., and Costigliola, P. (1993a). 'Deliberate HIV infections, a way of committing suicide', *Italian Journal of Suicidology*, 1, p. 161.

Lazzari, C., and Costigliola, P. (1993b). *Sex and AIDS: Can the Sexual Transmission of AIDS Be Stopped?* Bologna: Pitagora University Library – Italy.

Lazzari, C., and Masino, M.A. (2015). *Psicologia e Filosofia della Salute* [Psychology and philosophy of health]. Milan: Libreriauniversitaria.it

Lazzari, C., Nikolou-Walker, E., and Liu, L. (2025). 'Self-Reflective Practice, Autoethnography, Storytelling, and Critical Incident Analysis in Exploratory Nursing and Midwifery Research: Facing Social Illnesses and Borderline Personality Disorder', *Iranian Journal of Nursing and Midwifery Research*, 30(3), pp. 413–420. doi: 10.4103/ijnmr.ijnmr_5_24

Lazzari, C., and Rabottini, M. (2022a). 'COVID-19, loneliness, social isolation and risk of dementia in older people: a systematic review and meta-analysis of the relevant literature', *International Journal of Psychiatry in Clinical Practice*, 26(2), pp. 196–207.

Lazzari, C., and Rabottini, M. (2022b). 'Samos syndrome, borderline personality disorder and Pathophilia: Why we cannot stop pandemics', *International Journal of Psychiatry Research*, 4(2), 22–26.

Lazzari, C., and Rabottini, M. (2024a). 'Persons with borderline personality disorder and pathophilia: Understanding causes of pandemic diffusion of transmissible diseases through Samos Syndrome', *European Psychiatry*, 67(S1). Available from: https://www.cambridge.org/core/journals/european-psychiatry/study/persons-with-borderline-personality-disorder-and-pathophilia-understanding-causes-of-pandemic-diffusion-of-transmissible-diseases-through-samos-syndrome/831C4BA8ACA3E094B1C82E78F9121434 [Accessed: 24 September 2025].

Lazzari, C., and Rabottini, M. (2024b). 'Socially ill: the new generation of medical and psychiatric patients', *Minerva Psych*, 65(2), pp.250–252.

Lazzari, C., and Rabottini, M. (2025a). 'Human Behaviors and Social Dynamics in Primary Prevention Failures During Pandemics: A Narrative Review of Behavioral and Systemic Challenges in Primary Prevention', *Disease and Health: Research Developments*, 6, pp. 54–89.

Lazzari, C., and Rabottini, M. (2025b). *Psychosocial Dynamics and Behavioural Compliance in Pandemic Response*. IGI Global. Available from: https://www.igi-global.com/book/psychosocial-dynamics-pandemic-response/312944

Lazzari, C., et al. (1996). 'Neurocognitive effects of Zidovudine and 2', 3'-Dideoxyinosine during the treatment of asymptomatic and symptomatic HIV-1 seropositive patients. Comparison with non-treated patients', *Human Psychopharmacology: Clinical and Experimental*, 11(5), pp. 415–420.

Lazzari, C., et al. (2023). 'Samos Syndrome, persons with borderline personality disorder and risk for sexually transmitted infections and HIV: Their role during pandemics', *Current Innovations in Disease and Health Research*, 7, pp. 12–21.

Lazzari, C., Campione, F., Mariani, L., Costigliola, P., Ricchi, E., and Chiodo, F. (1991). *La Sindrome di Samos* [The syndrome of Samos]. Presented at the National Congress of the Italian Society of Psychiatry, Salsomaggiore Terme, Italy, October 1991.

Lazzari, C., Costigliola, P., Di Bari, M.A., De Ronchi, D., Volterra, V., and Chiodo, F. (1994). 'AIDS has an increasing diffusion within the heterosexual population', *AIDS Patient Care*, 8(3), p. 106.

Lazzari, C., Costley, C., and Nikolou-Walker, E. (2024). *Interprofessional and Intraprofessional Teamwork and Handovers in Healthcare: Challenges and Recommendations from Work-based Learning*. Faringdon: Libri Publishing.

Lazzari, C., Gandolfi Colleoni, G., and Trallo, F. (1996). *Eros. Malattie sessuali. Società* [Eros, sexual diseases and society]. Bologna: Pitagora Editrice.

Lazzari, C., McAleer, S., Nusair, A., and Rabottini, M. (2021). 'Psychiatric training during the COVID-19 pandemic benefits from integrated practice in interprofessional teams and ecological momentary e-assessment', *Rivista di Psichiatria*, 56(2), pp. 74–84.

Lazzari, C., McAleer, S., and Rabottini, M. (2022). 'The assessment of interprofessional practice in mental health nursing with ethnographic observation and social network analysis: A confirmatory and exploratory mixed-methods study', *Rivista di Psichiatria*, 57(5), pp. 246–254.

Lazzari, C., Nusair, A., Shoka, A., Hein, S.M., and Rabottini, M. (2020a). 'Case reports of first psychiatric presentations during COVID-19 pandemic', *Rivista di Psichiatria*, 55(5), pp. 319–321.

Lazzari, C., Nusair, A., Shoka, A., and Rabottini, M. (2020b). 'Psychiatry During COVID-19 Pandemic: A Case Report of Attempted Mercy Killing', *Psychiatria Danubina*, 32(2), pp. 303–304.

Lazzari, C., Rees, J., Graham, Y., and Owens, R. (2025). 'Psychiatric comorbidities and sexual health risks in HIV-serodiscordant hetero-sexual couples involving women with borderline personality disorder: A mixed-methods study and theoretical modeling', *Preprints*, 3 December. doi: 10.20944/preprints202512.0374.v1.

Lazzari, C., Shoka, A., Nusair, A., Hein, S.M., and Rabottini, M. (2020c). 'Clinical psychopathology during COVID-19 pandemic: case reports of first psychiatric presentations', *Psychiatria Danubina*, 32(Suppl. 4), pp. 597–601.

Lazzari, C., Shoka, A., Nusair, A., and Rabottini, M. (2020d). 'Psychiatry in Time of COVID-19 Pandemic', *Psychiatria Danubina*, 32(2), pp. 229–235.

Lazzari, C., Shoka, A., Papanna, B., and Rabottini, M. (2018). 'The hypothesis of a tripolar syndrome in liaison psychiatry and medicine: Depression comorbid with factitious disorders and borderline personality disorder', *Indian Journal of Medical Research and Pharmaceutical Science*, 5(4), pp. 61–68.

Lehman, B.J., David, D.M., and Gruber, J.A. (2017). 'Rethinking the biopsychosocial model of health: Understanding health as a dynamic system', *Social and Personality Psychology Compass*, 11(8).

Lehrer, K. (1990). *Theory of Knowledge*. 2nd edn. Boulder, CO: Westview Press.

Lin, H. (2007). 'Knowledge sharing and firm innovation capability: an empirical study', *International Journal of Manpower*, 28(3/4), pp. 315–332.

Lincoln, Y.S., and Guba, E.G. (1985). *Naturalistic Inquiry*. Newbury Park, CA: SAGE Publications.

Liu, W., and Liu, J. (2021). 'Living with COVID-19: A phenomenological study of hospitalised patients' experiences'. *BMJ Open*, 11(2), e046128.

Liu, Y., Zhang, H., and Wang, X. (2023). 'Sensory impairments and social isolation in middle-aged and older adults in China', *BMC Geriatrics*, 23(1), pp. 112–125.

Liu, C.H., Zhang, E., Wong, G.T.F., Hyun, S., and Hahm, H.C. (2021). 'Factors associated with depression, anxiety, and PTSD symptomatology during the COVID19 pandemic: a clinical study of young adults', *Journal of Affective Disorders*, 281, pp. 230–237.

Lowe, A., Voo, T., Lee, L., et al. (2022). 'Uncertainty, scarcity and transparency: Public health ethics and risk communication in a pandemic', *The Lancet Regional Health – Americas*, 16, 100366. Available from: https://www.sciencedirect.com/science/article/pii/S2667193X22000732

Luchetti, M., Sutin, A.R., and Terracciano, A. (2022). 'A meta-analysis of loneliness and risk of dementia using longitudinal data', *Journal of Gerontology: Psychological Sciences*, 77(5), pp. 923–935.

Mahawar, K.K., Clare, K., O'Kane, M., Graham, Y., Callejas-Diaz, L., and Carr, W.R.J. (2019). 'Patient perspectives on adherence with micronutrient supplementation after bariatric surgery', *Obesity Surgery*, 29(5), pp. 1551–1556.

Mahesar, A., Shah, S.A., Shaikh, S., and Mahesar, R. (2023). 'Psychiatric implications of COVID19 lockdown and suicide reporting in Pakistani media: a content analysis', *Pakistan Journal of Medical Sciences*, 39(1), pp. 250–256.

Malterud, K. (2001). 'Qualitative research: standards, challenges, and guidelines', *The Lancet*, 358(9280), pp. 483–488.

Marmot, M., and Wilkinson, R.G. (2006). *Social Determinants of Health*. 2nd edn. Oxford: Oxford University Press.

Martin, P., de Saille, S., Liddiard, K., and Pearce, W. (eds.) (2022). *Being Human During COVID-19*. Bristol: Bristol University Press.

Matić, I., Takšić, V., and Božičević, S. (2021). 'Emotional competence and resilience during concurrent crises: psychological responses to earthquakes and the COVID19 pandemic in Croatia', *Current Psychology*, 40(12), pp. 5900–5912.

McClimans, L.M. (2024). *Patient-Centered Measurement: Ethics, Epistemology, and Dialogue in Contemporary Medicine.* Oxford: Oxford University Press.

McCrory, E.J., Gerin, M.I., and Viding, E. (2017). 'Annual Research Review: Childhood maltreatment, latent vulnerability and the shift to preventative psychiatry – the contribution of functional brain imaging', *Journal of Child Psychology and Psychiatry,* 58(4), pp. 338–357.

Merleau-Ponty, M. (1962). *Phenomenology of Perception.* London: Routledge and Kegan Paul.

Merriam-Webster (2024). 'Solipsism'. Oakland: Merriam-Webster, Incorporated. Available from: https://www.merriam-webster.com/dictionary/solipsism [Accessed: 30 October 2025].

Merriam-Webster Dictionary (2025). 'Pandemic'. Available from: https://www.merriam-webster.com/dictionary/pandemic [Accessed: 21 September 2025].

Monteith, S., Glenn, T., Geddes, J.R., Whybrow, P.C., and Bauer, M. (2021). 'Digital psychiatry in the aftermath of COVID19: the rise of online risks and cybervulnerability', *The Lancet Psychiatry,* 8(7), pp. 633–640.

Nandy, M., Lodh, S., and Tang, A. (2021). 'Lessons from COVID-19 and a resilience model for higher education', *Industry and Higher Education,* 35(1), pp. 3–9.

NHS (2024). *Consent to Treatment – Assessing Capacity.* London: National Health Service. Available from: https://www.nhs.uk/tests-and-treatments/consent-to-treatment/capacity/ [Accessed: 16 April 2026].

NHS England (2023). *A National Framework for NHS Action on Inclusion Health.* Available from: https://www.england.nhs.uk/long-read/a-national-framework-for-nhs-action-on-inclusion-health/

Nie, J., Zhang, Y., and Li, X. (2021). 'Behavioral inconsistency in public health compliance during COVID-19', *Social Behaviour and Health,* 9(2), pp. 88–97.

Owens, R., Blagden, N., Winder, B., Hegarty, K., and Farias, M. (2021). 'Changes in sexual desire and behaviors among UK young adults during social lockdown due to COVID-19', *The Journal of Sex Research,* 58(8), pp. 983–993.

Pears, R., and Shields, G. (2019). *Cite Them Right: The Essential Referencing Guide.* 11th edn. London: Macmillan.

Plato (2007). *The Republic*. London: Penguin Classics.

Pretorius, L. (2024). 'Demystifying research paradigms: navigating ontology, epistemology, and axiology in research', *The Qualitative Report*, 29(10), pp. 2698–2715.

Prommas, P., Chen, Y., and Lin, M. (2023). 'The impact of social isolation from COVID-19 on cognitive function and mental health among older adults', *Geriatrics and Gerontology International*, 23(3), pp. 210–222.

Pronk, N.P., Woodard, C., Zimmerman, F.J., and Arena, R. (2025). 'An ecological framework for population health and well-being', *Progress in Cardiovascular Diseases*, 90 (May–June), pp. 13–21.

Psicologi Italia (2025). *La Sindrome di Samo*. Available from: https://www.psicologi-italia.it/disturbi-e-terapie/psicoterapia/articoli/la-sindrome-di-samo.html

Public Health England (2020). *National COVID19 Surveillance Reports*. London: Public Health England. Available from: https://www.gov.uk/government/publications/national-covid-19-surveillance-reports (gov.uk in Bing) [Accessed: 3 February 2026].

Rania, N., and Coppola, I. (2021). 'Psychological impact of the COVID19 outbreak on Italian university students: changes in mental health and lifestyle', *International Journal of Environmental Research and Public Health*, 18(17), 9420.

Raw, R.K., Rees, J., Kelly, C.A., Wroe, C., and Chadwick, D.R. (2022). 'Prior COVID-19 infection is associated with increased Adverse Events (AEs) after the first, but not the second, dose of the BNT162b2/Pfizer vaccine', *Vaccine*, 40(3), pp. 418–423.

Rittmannsberger, H., Barth, M., Malik, P., Malsiner-Walli, G., and Yazdi, K. (2022). 'First-episode psychotic disorders in the wake of the COVID-19 pandemic: A descriptive review of case reports', *Acta Neuropsychiatrica*, 34(6), pp. 317–329.

Ritunnano, R., Papola, D., Broome, M.R., and Nelson, B. (2023). 'Phenomenology as a Resource for Translational Research in Mental Health', *Epidemiology and Psychiatric Sciences*, 32.

Sayeed, A., Kundu, S., Al Banna, M.H., Christopher, E., Hasan, M.T., Begum, M.R., and Khan, M.S.I. (2020). 'Mental health outcomes of adults with chronic diseases during the COVID19 pandemic: a crosssectional study', *BMC Psychiatry*, 20, 489.

Schwandt, T.A. (2007). *The Sage Dictionary of Qualitative Inquiry*. 3rd edn. Thousand Oaks, CA: Sage.

Scotland, J. (2012). 'Exploring the conceptual underpinnings of research: Relating ontology and epistemology to the methodology and methods of the scientific, interpretive, and critical research paradigms', *English Language Teaching*, 5(9), pp. 9–16.

Sehlikoğlu, Ş., and Almiş, B.H. (2022). 'First episode psychosis following COVID-19 infection: two case reports from Turkey', *Psychiatry and Behavioral Sciences*, 12(2), p. 94.

Smith, B. (2019). *Ontology and the Epistemology of Health*. Buffalo: SUNY Press.

Smith, M. (2020). 'It really does depend: Towards an epistemology (and ontology) for everyday social pedagogical practice', *International Journal of Social Pedagogy*, 9(1), pp. 1–18.

Stewart, D., and Mikunas, A. (1974). *Exploring Phenomenology: A Guide to the Field and Its Literature*. Athens: Ohio University Press.

Strauss, A., and Corbin, J. (1990). *Basics of Qualitative Research: Grounded Theory Procedures and Techniques*. Newbury Park, CA: Sage Publications.

Svenaeus, F. (2001). 'The hermeneutics of medicine and the phenomenology of health', *Medicine, Health Care and Philosophy*, 4(3), pp. 285–294.

Teo, D.C.H., Choo, X.Y., and Tang, C.T. (2024). 'The first reported case of new-onset mania and psychosis post heterologous bivalent mRNA COVID-19 booster vaccination', *Psychiatry Research Case Reports*, 3(1), pp. 17–21.

Thompson, A.K., and Upshur, R.E.G. (2017). 'Justice and vulnerability in pandemic ethics', *Public Health Ethics*, 10(1), pp. 1–9.

Todorov, M., Avramova-Todorova, G., and Bureva, V. (2023). 'Emotional intelligence of students during pandemic outbreak: A study in higher education', in *Recent Trends in Data Science and Soft Computing*. Springer, pp. 246–257.

UK Health Security Agency (2025). *National Flu and COVID-19 Surveillance Report: 16 October 2025 (week 42).* Available from: https://www.gov.uk/government/statistics/national-flu-and-Covid-19-surveillance-reports-2025-to-2026-season/national-flu-and-Covid-19-surveillance-report-16-october-2025-week-42 [Accessed: 27 October 2025].

Upshur, R.E. (2002). 'Principles for the justification of public health intervention', *Canadian Journal of Public Health*, 93(2), pp. 101–103.

Usul, E., Şan, İ., and Bekgöz, B. (2020). 'The effect of the COVID19 pandemic on anxiety levels of emergency medical service workers', *Journal of Emergency Medicine Case Reports*, 11(4), pp. 126–130.

Valli, R., Luzi, A.M., Bianconi, M., Camoni, L., Colucci, A., Frati, A., Gallo, P., Rosa, E., and D'Agostini, A. (2002). *La prevenzione dell'infezione da HIV, i giovani e le loro conoscenze: un'indagine su un campione di adolescenti italiani* [HIV prevention, young people and their knowledge: a survey of Italian adolescents]. *Annali dell'Istituto Superiore di Sanità*, 38(4), pp. 377–386.

van Manen, M. (1990). *Researching Lived Experience: Human Science for an Action Sensitive Pedagogy*. Albany, NY: SUNY Press.

Visvizi, A., Nawaz, R., and Kozłowski, K. (eds.) (2023). *Higher Education Institutions and COVID-19: Toward Resilience and Sustainability through Emergencies*. Routledge.

WHO (World Health Organization) (2020). *Strengthening Community Protection and Resilience for Health Emergencies*. Geneva: WHO. Available from: https://www.who.int/activities/strengthening-community-readiness-for-health-emergencies [Accessed: 8 April 2026].

WHO (World Health Organization) (2021). 'Pandemic Definition' – Public Health. Available from: https://www.publichealth.com.ng/world-health-organization-who-pandemic-definition/

WHO (World Health Organization) (2023). *Infection Prevention and Control in the Context of COVID-19: A Guideline*. Geneva: WHO. Available from: https://www.who.int/publications/i/item/WHO-2019-nCoV-IPC-guideline-2023.4

WHO (World Health Organization) (2025). *What Are Critical Incidents?* Work Positive. Available from: https://www.workpositive.ie/node/1905

Watts (1999). Epidemics and History: Disease, Power and Imperialism. London: Routledge.

Wikipedia Contributors (2023). *Sindrome di Samo*. Available from: https://it.wikipedia.org/wiki/Sindrome_di_Samo

World Medical Association (2022). *Declaration of Helsinki: Ethical Principles for Medical Research Involving Human Subjects*. Available from: https://www.wma.net/policies-post/wma-declaration-of-helsinki-ethical-principles-for-medical-research-involving-human-subjects/

Yasin, A., and AlTamimi, A. (2020). 'Fear of COVID19 and psychological distress in the general population: the role of cognitive framing', *Journal of Community Psychology*, 48(8), pp. 2850–2862.

Yilmaz, M., Erdogan, A., and Bahadir, E. (2021). 'Burnout, sleep problems and psychological distress among frontline healthcare workers during the COVID19 pandemic', *Journal of Clinical Nursing*, 30(21–22), pp. 3200–3210.

Zahavi, D., and Szanto, T. (2023). 'Emotions of the pandemic: Phenomenological perspectives', *Phenomenology and the Cognitive Sciences*, 22(1), pp. 1–15.

Zambaco Pacha (1981). *Voyage chez les lépreux*. Paris: Éditions L'Harmattan.

www.ingramcontent.com/pod-product-compliance
Lightning Source LLC
LaVergne TN
LVHW050917210926
848482LV00012B/470
* 9 7 8 1 9 1 1 4 5 1 4 9 5 *